NATURE WALKING WITH CANCER

Also by Dr. Randy Kidd

Dr. Kidd's Guide to Herbal Cat Care (2000), Storey Publishing.
Dr. Kidd's Guide to Herbal Dog Care (2000), Storey Publishing.

NATURE WALKING WITH CANCER

REUNITING THE HUMAN SPIRIT WITH THE SOUL OF NATURE

Randy Kidd, D.V.M., Ph.D.

Anamcara Press LLC
Lawrence, Kansas

Published in 2024 by Anamcara Press LLC
Author © 2024 by Randy Kidd, D.V.M., Ph.D.
Cover design by Morgan Shaw, Randy's Granddaughter-in-law
Palitino Linotype, Minion Pro, Trebuchet, Chealsea Market Pro
Printed in the United States of America.
Book description: Nature Walking with Cancer advocates embracing life with both
hands through activity, nature, creativity, and love, offering a fresh perspective
on terminal illness and inspiring readers to live fully despite a cancer diagnosis.

The poem "Tide" reprinted with permission from the author, H C Palmer
https://www.feet-of-the-messenger.com.

ANAMCARA PRESS LLC
P.O. Box 442072, Lawrence, KS 66044
https://anamcara-press.com

Ordering Information:
Quantity sales. Special discounts are available on quantity purchases by corpo-
rations, associations, and others. For details, contact the publisher at the address
above. Orders by U.S. trade bookstores and wholesalers. Please contact Ingram
Distribution.

ISBN-13: Nature Walking With Cancer, 978-1-960462-50-3 (Paperback)
ISBN-13: Nature Walking With Cancer, 978-1-960462-52-7 (EBook)
ISBN-13: Nature Walking With Cancer, 978-1-960462-51-0 (Hardcover)
HEA039030 HEALTH & FITNESS / Diseases & Conditions / Cancer
HEA015000 HEALTH & FITNESS / Men's Health
OCC043000 BODY, MIND & SPIRIT / Nature Therapy
SPO050000 SPORTS & RECREATION / Walking
TP060   TOPICAL / Health & Fitness
TP064   TOPICAL / Inspiration
Library of Congress Control Number: 2024939709

CONTENTS

PART ONE: In The Beginning

Diagnosis

I

Diagnosis (June 2018): "I am so sorry to tell you this," she begins, her voice cracking as she speaks, "but you have Stage 4 prostate cancer."

So that's what all this has been about, I'm thinking. A couple of months ago I had vague back pains that a cadre of "docs" had tried to diagnose, using a host of different diagnostic tools, without much luck. The pain persisted and I noticed some numbness in my chest and feet … but hell, I'm 76 years old and a lot of my body parts have gone numb on me.

My wife Sue and I continued to walk our two miles almost every day until Thursday. On Friday, the legs were too numb for walking, so we set up another trip to the doctor's office for the following week. Saturday I had complete Jell-O legs, and our calls to the doc on Monday moved us into an emergency MRI exam set up for late Wednesday night; the earliest there was a slot available.

Thursday morning, after the MRI, we are called into the doctor's office and ushered into the conference room/lunchroom for a talk with Nurse Amy. Nurse Amy is one of those young, bubbly personalities who makes you believe that all the world's ills are still capable of being fixed. Thursday is the morning when Nurse Amy gave us her "I'm so sorry, but" speech.

My first thought: OK, so this is not all that scary, no big whoop – at least according to what I'd read about prostate cancer in older men. At my age almost all prostatic cancers are so slow growing you will die of old age before the cancer gets you. Turns out I'd neglected to read the fine print.

The fine print: A small percentage of prostate cancers – mostly depending on the genetics involved – have the tendency to develop into more severe, metastatic, cancers. Later, much later, I will delve further into the fine print … and learn that I am one of the lucky ones to have at least four of the gene sequences that predispose me to developing the nasty, terminal kind of metastatic prostate cancer ... and several more that may also be problem children.

Nurse Amy says we need to go directly to the emergency room (ER) at Lawrence Memorial Hospital (LMH). She looks away while offering me a hug and I feel that none of this augurs well as omen for my future.

II

Emergency Room: Sue drives me to the emergency room. We sit there waiting for the ambulance. The ER Doc comes in, explains that the MRI showed the cancer has spread from my prostate into other parts of my body. One tumor is growing into my spinal canal, pushing my spinal cord to the side. This tumor is the likely cause of my legs going numb.

"We're sending you to Kansas University Med Center for further evaluation," he says. "It's likely they'll have to do surgery." Our ER doc is old and fatherly. He says he's sorry to tell me this. Says it's never easy. Says that's part of the reason he'll be retiring soon. He does not hug me. He leaves the room and quietly shuts the door.

Sue and I don't speak; don't look at each other. What does one think about in moments like these? The tile on the floor is well-worn, well-scrubbed; the walls a dirty off-white with the paint peeling in one corner. Our seats are hospital-issue: lined up against the wall, wooden arm rests, padded seats covered in black plastic that is cracked in several places – I'm thinking they could use a good dose of duct tape. The room is eerily quiet.

The quiet gives the mind the space to begin what will become a long line of questions: What did I do to deserve this? What could I have done to avoid it? I've been living a holistically healthy lifestyle ... and yet there's this, this cancer eating at my innards, gnawing on my teeth and bones, swallowing my soul. I want to ask: "Why me God? Why me?" ... even though none of the God-guy religions have ever been a part of my belief system.

Sitting there in the quiet, I am not getting answers; only questions. What now? What next?

In the quiet I am revisited by a nagging dream I've been having, off and on, for several months now.

III

The Dream: The head of a snake appears from under the covers as I sleep. This snake seems like a friendly snake. Is that a mischievous grin I see as his head edges toward my pillow? It is only when his nose begins to nudge my neck that I realize how huge he is.

I feel the scaley-chill of reptile slither over my body. One loop coiled around my chest. I can feel the weight of the snake pressing me down; the coil wraps tighter. Thin slits of his black pupils glare directly into my eyes. He rears back with mouth open wide. It is a huge mouth, long glistening-white fangs pointed forward, aimed at my shoulder.

It is a flash of snake-strike that hits my left shoulder – the one that I haven't been able to lift since the wear and tear of college football ruined it many years ago. Although he is lightning fast, the strike seems to be almost playful – as if toying with me.

His fangs are needle sharp as they meet my shoulder bones. It is a strike of surgical accuracy; I flinch away from the biting pain of fangs. Is that me moaning as I feel the dull, throb-like pain of him chewing on my shoulder to assure maximum poison release? Or is it the moan of a ghost in the room?

The pain of the bite disappears as quickly as it was administered. The snake seems to be gently massaging my shoulder as he finishes injecting his poison. He releases his hold on my shoulder, and then, in some of the dreams, he opens his mouth wide, just to show me the size of his maw – wide enough to swallow my head whole if he wanted to. In other dreams he seems to be chuckling, a wicked grin on his face, as he quickly disappears from sight under my covers.

This final mockery is what wakes me, lying in a pool of sweat.

All this happens much faster than I can write the words to describe it. I've interpreted my dream snake to be a bushmaster, Lachesis muta, the largest venomous snake in the Western Hemisphere.

But, because I can only remember a few things about him -- his huge size, the viperine slant of his pupils, the death-like fixation of eye-gaze, the huge heat-sensing pits just below his nostrils, and those long ivory-white fangs -- I don't have him positively identified.

IV

Last Words: My dreams are so vivid in their symbolism, I should have been able to easily interpret them. Was it Jung who claimed that dreams should be difficult to interpret because interpretations require really knowing the dreamer? (Or was it Freud who said that? Or John Wayne?)

The only thing clear to me now is that I don't really know me – at least the new me, the me who has cancer. A new me, with or without dreams.

Chapter One: Interlude

I

Homeopathic Constitutional Remedies: During my homeopathic training, several homeopathic practitioners diagnosed my constitutional remedy as Lachesis. Homeopaths believe that the correct constitutional remedy to treat a patient can be determined by observing the totality of the patient's symptoms – physical, mental, and emotional.

Symptoms that correlate with the Lachesis diagnosis as my "constitutional" remedy include: 1) physical: A lot of left-sided conditions (my dysfunctional left shoulder, as but one example); 2) mental: a mind that often becomes crowded with thoughts; and 3) emotional: easily aggravated into aggressive behaviors.

These symptoms I remember. They are, after all, an ongoing part of the inner me.

With this in mind, I've always thought the snaky dreams were sent to me to remind me to use Lachesis remedy to work toward healing my bad shoulder. But, after dosing with the Lachesis remedy, the shoulder would get slightly better for a week or two … then continue to get worse.

Perhaps the snake was symbolic of something else. Or perhaps my dream snake was not Lachesis after all – perhaps he was symbolic of a rattlesnake or a copperhead, both of which I've actually met up with in the wilds.

II

The Fates: But there is a different symbology of Lachesis, and it is now the new me, the me with cancer, the me sitting, thinking in the ER room, waiting for the ambulance, that remembers *this* Lachesis. It is Lachesis – along with her sisters Atropos and Clotho – who is one of the mythological Three Fates in ancient Greek religion.

The Fates (also known as Moirai) were responsible in some way for determining a person's fate or destiny in life, and how they did this was related to the spinning of cloth. One of the Fates spun the "cloth of life"; another measured its length, deciding how long life should be; and the third cut the cloth (as a metaphor for death).

My problem now, waiting in the Emergency Room, is that I can't remember which of the Fates Lachesis represents: the spinner, the measurer, or "now's the time to whack it off" Fate.

III

Last Words: Struggling with this question, the ER crew that is to take me to the KC hospital arrives. And so, it looks like I will be stuck with the image of the Three Fates spinning the fate of my life from now on, one of them ultimately cutting their spun cloth … to end my life.

Code Talkers

The Ambulance: I am now lying on the ambulance stretcher, appropriately stretched out and strapped down. My two thoughts, as they were wheeling me, headfirst, through the double doored portal to the innards of the ambulance: 1) Jonah and the whale, and 2) the jaws of a huge constrictor snake that can – due to its unique construction that combines loosely connected jaw bones and stretchy, elasticized ligaments and skin – open its maw wide enough to swallow my entire head.

I am reminded of the contrast between parable and reality as the doors to the ambulance are swung wide to allow for the gulping of me and my stretcher. Trying to sort out these two stories – Nature's mythology from its reality – confuses me.

Perhaps I will, like Jonah, be resurrected from my death sentence. Or will my fate be to lie within the belly of a huge constrictor? Who knows?

My ride will be taking me from the emergency room at LMH to KU Med, Kansas University's hospital complex located in KC, 30-some miles down the highway. This is about the only thing I am certain of. This and the fact that an EMT (Emergency Medical Technician) sits next to me in the ambulance, clipboard in hand.

Once settled into the ambulance, I am asked yet again to repeat my name, my birth date, and on a scale of 1 to 10 how much pain I'm feeling; and finally, do I feel safe at home. Trying to change the subject. I ask how fast we are going. "About 80 mph," I'm told. "That's normal for these kinds of runs." I can feel the coils of my restraints tightening around my chest; there is a sharp pain, penetrating my spine where the tumor is growing. I look heavenward for signs of divine intervention – seeing only the roof of an ambulance.

II

Code Talkers: This run is what in EMT lingo is called a non-emergent run – I'm just being hauled from one place to another. I know this because I've been a Volunteer Fireman/First Responder for Sarcoxie Township, a small rural fire department just north of Lawrence, Kansas.

One of your early lessons as a first responder is that Med-Speak is done in codes, as in non-emergent. The second thing you learn is that there are perhaps a gazillion codes: codes for firemen, cops, medical personnel, first responders, private pilots; commercial aviators, air force pilots, drug dealers, deaf people, deaf people who are drug dealers, and on and on. Thirdly, each district – country, state, city, village, county, or township -- has its own coding system. And finally, none of the coding systems communicate very well, if at all, with any of the others.

Since this ambulance run originated in one county south of where I'd been a first responder, our coding on this run will likely be something different from what I'd learned. Instead of non-emergent, perhaps this county refers to it as a *Code-Green* or a *10-37* (both of which are code for "nonemergency, no sirens"). I'm pretty sure that I have not yet reached the Code Black category (the category for: We are carrying a patient who is Obviously Dead, and so we will not be using our siren or lights).

III

Portals: The gist of all this is that I have passed through the portals of entry into the Wonderful World of Medicine – more specifically, I have passed through the portals of entry into the Wonderful World of **Western** Medicine or even more specifically yet, into the Wonderful World of **Western Oncology** Medicine.

As I begin my pilgrimage through the portals that lead into that sacred kingdom of cancer medicine, wishing I had Toto riding alongside, perhaps gnawing at the restraining straps on my stretcher, I will learn there is also a coding of all the systems of medicine in this country, including a lengthy coding for oncology (cancer medicine) and the indecipherable coding for how your oncology treatment bills must be paid.

At every turn along the way I will be reminded that all this coding is incredibly baffling – even for someone like me who has lived with it as a part of my veterinary career. I will come to believe that, in fact, it is *meant* to be baffling – baffling to the point of being disturbingly clownish.

Maybe I'll just laugh when they present me with my bill.

IV

Power Hungry: My mind wanders as we jostle along an eroding and pock-marked I-70 -- Eisenhower's highway system to ensure his tanks could, in case of war, move with due speed from one part of the country to another. I know now that a horde of invading cancer cells has taken over my body and laid siege on it, intent on blasting my bones into bits and then devouring the fragments.

War as metaphor works particularly well for the now I am in, strapped onto a stretcher, bouncing along a made-for-war highway, headed toward a battlefield-type surgery that will take out only the biggest chunk of the main projectile of my cancer, leaving behind a scattering of smaller bits of tumorous shrapnel. The malignant shards of shrapnel will remain embedded in tissue and continue to cause pain and misery as they march ever onward, destroying tissues wherever they go.

Were he to be commander of the malignant cells now infecting my body, Civil War General, Wm. Tecumseh Sherman, would be proud of his troops, and perhaps I should start to think of my metastatic cancer cells as being engaged in a "scorched earth" policy as they make their way through my body, ala Gen. Sherman's March to the Sea.

The initial battlefield has been set by the suddenness of the attack, and I am beholden (for now) to the corps of medical resources that will be made available to me: the battlefield surgeons. I understand that I have ceded all the power over my body to the god-like system of Western Medicine. As a practitioner who has used many forms of medicine, and as a person who wants to believe he is always in control, the ceding of power to "another" is not a comfortable feeling.

I look out the back window of the ambulance and see the cars and semis pulled over to give way to our blinking red, white and blue lights. I am thinking that perhaps, just maybe, I might still have some power left in me after all. Feeling that smidgen of joy juice, I want more. I ask if they could possibly, please, turn the siren on. "That's not protocol," a gruff voice replies. (I assume that using a siren on this type of run must then be a Code *10-30 – against policy*).

V

Man Power: Leaving behind the thought of any iota of power remaining within, my thoughts turn to another worry, silently gnawing at the very core of my essence. When a dog is diagnosed with prostate cancer or even when he has an age-related (and almost always benign) enlarged prostate, we veterinarians castrate him. It's considered good practice. "Probably should have been done earlier," we say. "That would have prevented the swelling of his prostate, and his nighttime dribbling, and he'd be fine." And we'd be done with it.

Don't get me wrong. I'm not, Lord knows I am definitely not, saying they should have castrated me at an earlier age. But, as we ride along, I am wondering how they plan to treat my cancer after they remove that one troublesome tumor. I can also visualize all those critters – dogs, cats, pigs, horses, cattle, and more – that I've castrated, each and every one of them tugging at their leash or rolling over in his grave, now silently rejoicing: "Cut him doc!" they sing in unison. "Take his balls out, just like he took ours. Let him see how it feels. Do it now!"

Ah, but we shall see.

I already know that my own testicles have something to do with the cancer I have – testosterone is the driving force behind prostate cancers, in both dogs and men. I also realize that something will need to be done with those infernal testosterone producers, my precious cajones. In my head, I assume that Western Medicine's oncology has surely come up with some magic bullet to knock-out my testosterone production.

So, it will come as a bit of a surprise when my oncologist, during our first visit, wants to know if I would accept being castrated. "It's a simple five-minute operation," he will explain.

Without thinking, I answer: "Not for me doc," I say. "I am way too fond of fondling them."

VI

Last Words: And so, one could ask the question: When faced with the prospect of death … or of maintaining his own vanity, why is it that the male of our species (me included) so often opts to keep his vanity?

One could also ask why the mind tends to become a storyteller in times such as these: riding in the ambulance to an unknown fate, wanting to – in any way possible – lighten the moment?

Why is it that my mind, in particular, wanders to a long-ago story that still carries its own brand of humor, albeit a brand of humor mostly reserved for veterinarians?

Chapter 2 Interlude: Castrating Pigs

Introduction: There's no finer way to take power away from an animal than to castrate him. A castrated animal is more docile, easier to handle, less aggressive … and fits more easily into the farmer's ideal of maintaining his own power so he can generate cash more easily and more effectively.

I'm thinking about all this as we are careening down Eisenhower's Road, red, white, and blue lights blinking overhead, with no siren sound – on a non-emergent (Code-Green or 19-37) run.

I'm trying to apply my thinking about what will be happening to me as I will likely be subjected to cancer therapy drugs that will effectively castrate me, when … when a very strange story out of the past comes to mind. Me thinks it is the Irish in me, responsible for these strange interludes of thought that come out of nowhere.

II

Cutting pigs was always one of my favorite things to do as a mixed-animal veterinarian. Put on boots, scrub boots so farmer knows you are trying to be clean, go to the pig sty or hog barn with scalpel (specially curved for its function as a castrator) soaking in a wash bucket containing disinfectant, and multidose vaccine syringes (if needed).

And don't forget that save-it basin. The save-it basin is for the testicles, which I will typically share with the farmer – we will clean those vittles and eat 'em later. Yum, yum. Nut fries: a Kansas treat.

As you walk to the surgery site, you hope your hog catchers and holders are brutishly big and strong. You also hope each of the pigs destined for surgery weighs less than 100 pounds.

One day, I decide to show Sue what fun it is to spend a few hours in the muck of hog manure, cutting young piglets. It's the neighbor's pigs, so I probably won't even charge them for the job, and they already know Sue. So, Sue and I pack up and head down the road.

Farmer and son are waiting for us, as are a couple dozen pigs wallowing around in a muddy pen behind the hog barn. The pigs are of all sizes and ages, from about 15 to 20 pounds to at least 100 pounds. I tell farmer and son that Sue is along to see how much fun this could be, and farmer immediately offers with a grin: "Well then, she needs to get out there and catch a few pigs herself, just to see what that's like."

Thinking that this could prove interesting, I loan her my boots and tell her to have at it.

Sue and farmer's son slog out, and Sue tries to catch her first pig ... which runs away, squealing. Sue, being a fast learner, quickly realizes the squealers need to be pinned against a fence corner, so you can grab a leg.

Sue pins a small piglet, reaches for and misses one leg, then another, tries again, reaches far out, loses one of my too-large boots which stays behind, sticking straight up in the mud. She turns to retrieve the boot, loses her balance, puts one hand down in muddy crud for balance, turns to reach for the boot, misses. She is now "three legged" – one bare hand, one bare foot, and one still-booted foot all mired in mud – spraddle-legged and looking to the sky for divine intervention.

I know this requires swift action. I set off on a dead run, scramble to get the car door open, fumble to retrieve the camera, and return as fast as I can for the perfect photo-op moment. Farmer and son are already at her side, trying to help, trying their best to keep from laughing, and not having much luck getting Sue upright... nor with keeping the laughter down.

I squeeze off a few snapshots before everything returns to near-normal. Sue glares at me as farmer and son wash off her bare foot and hand and other places where the muck splattered. I tell her she can dry off and watch from the car if she wants to.

In the veterinary trade we call these minor mishaps "wrecks," and we expect at least one wreck to happen whenever we work with livestock. Later, I will try to explain this to Sue, but now is probably not the time.

The rest of that day's pig cutting goes uneventfully. As I am packing up to leave, farmer calls me over, says with a huge grin: "Here, you take all the nuts. Having that wreck with Sue was sure worth it." It surely was.

I tried to find the photos of Sue stuck in the muck, but after looking high and low, they were nowhere to be found. Can't figure what might have happened to them. Shame too.

For those who have an insatiable appetite to learn more about cooking testicles, I have included more info on nut fries, Kansas style, in the notes following this chapter.

Notes: Chapter 2

Rocky Mountain Oysters: Bull testicles, in our area are usually known as Rocky Mountain oysters, but testicles on the menu may have any of several names: prairie oysters, cowboy caviar, Montana tendergroin, dusted nuts, swinging beef, bollocks, or simply mountain oysters. Pig, lamb, or turkey testicles are also menu fare, and are often referred to as pig/lamb/or turkey fries or nuts.

Health Benefits of Testicles: Testicles can be thought of as organ meat, rich in vitamins, minerals, and protein. While they are sometimes thought to be aphrodisiacs, animal testicles have no known effect on human hormones.

Tasty: Opinions vary, but most often the claim is that they "taste just like chicken, maybe a bit more chewy." Some folks think bull testicles have a slightly liver/gizzard flavor. One foodie commented that they were surprisingly "juicy", and others have said they have a slightly wild-game flavor.

Mountain Oyster Fixins, Easy-Peasy: Simply skin the outer cover off, cut in half (some folks also pound them to tenderize), dust with your favorite batter, and deep fat fry. Some of our locals first soak them overnight in baking soda, but I think that gives them an off taste. Others soak them in salt water for an hour and then parboil before they are fried, but I am too lazy for that (and I also think that takes away from their flavor). Still others might add their favorite spicy topping or cocktail sauce, but again, I prefer them simply breaded and fried.

Example recipe (for any nut fry: bull, lamb, pig, or turkey):

2 lbs. testicles – outer skin removed and testicles sliced into halves, lengthwise

2 tablespoons salt

1 cup flour

1/4 cup cornmeal

1 cup red wine (set aside the rest of the bottle... to help with digestion)

Flummoxed

I

Crisis Medicine: My castration reverie complete, I return, with an ironic grin, to where I am now – careening down I-70, headed for who knows what – hopefully not my own castration. As we ride along, I am thinking about another aspect of medicine, including veterinary medicine, that has always given me pause.

I've often wondered why it is that it takes a crisis to lift us off our lazy ass and get us to do anything that's good for our own health. To quit smoking, for example, or to exercise regularly, lose a few pounds, eat fewer of our favorite sugary desserts, sleep more regular hours, eat more of those anti-cancer veggies I keep meaning to read about so I'll know which ones are supposed to work.

Our human species seems bound and determined to keep on keeping on … right up to the day **the crisis** rears its ugly head. Then, and only then, do we decide to make those lifestyle choices that we knew to be healthy all along … if we are fortunate enough that **the crisis** hasn't killed us in the meantime.

As but one example: CDC data from 2019 shows that heart disease accounted for 659,041 deaths, and an additional 150,005 people died from strokes in the U.S. alone. Approximately 1.5 million heart attacks occur annually in the U.S. It has been estimated that 80% of the deaths from all forms of heart disease could be prevented … simply by changing some of our lifestyles.

According to CDC 2019 data, cancer takes another 599,601 lives a year, and most cancers are nudged into active mode by some dumbass habit we have – habits like: smoking or chewing tobacco, or drinking alcohol (or other toxic liquids), or rolling around in the pesticides and herbicides that make our lawns such beautiful places to behold, or working in a job (or living in an area) that exposes us to toxic levels of carcinogens.

Prostate cancer is one of the cancers that is a bit of an outlier here. Most prostate cancers are benign enough that they don't cause any real problems – it's said that if you're in your 60's or 70's when you get early-stage prostate cancer, you will die of old age before the cancer gets you.

The real cause of the typical prostate cancer is not really known. (I've been trying to convince my oncologist it's due to "overuse syndrome" … without much luck.) But, when the cells go rogue and decide to invade bones north and south of the prostate (i.e. when it becomes a Stage 4 cancer), the most likely cause is genetic. In my case, then, I guess *Tis the Luck o' the Irish a'Workin' On Me*…once again.

II

Coyote Cancer: All this is to say that this life-crisis, this time with *my* cancer, is different: My cancer has snuck up on us like a dark coyote in the black of the new moon. The "us" I refer to includes me and each one of several doctors who have been trying to diagnose the cause of my subtle and non-specific symptoms.

To be sure, I wasn't totally blindsided. I'd heard the soft paddling of coyote paws behind me and knew that I was being stalked. People who have the gut sense they are being stalked – stalked by a pair of coyotes, a pack of wolves, or a solo cougar – often report that it sends a chilling stab into the heart and makes the breath go quicker, flatter.

Then, when they backtrack on their trail, and when they see the actual tracks of the predator, following, and when those tracks confirm their worst fears, they often admit that the on-the-ground evidence of the stalker was almost a knock-out blow by itself – a punch to the gut that made their knees go weak and wobbly.

I know the feeling. My own stalker shot poison darts into my back, darts of pain that worsened and eventually kept me awake at night. Lying there, awake, I would try to backtrack my recent history, try to capture the evidence of my predator. I never saw identifiable spoor – only unexplained darkness, weirdness, sometimes scythes leaning against corn shocks or snakes slithering around, often the yellow moon-glare of unidentifiable eyes peering around the shocks, through the weeds. Staring, quietly glaring.

But, as I've said, I am old, mid-70's old, the age when almost all of us have back pains. What's more, I am wiser now, having been through a few life-crises already. And I am thinking that I can outsmart the predator, any predator, simply by doing due diligence, trying to figure out what might be happening and then doing something constructive about it.

Besides, I am armed. I am, after all, a veterinarian with a PhD in veterinary pathology. As a practitioner, for many years I used alternative medicines – acupuncture, herbals, chiropractic, homeopathy, and others. I know about disease, and I know the variety of medicines that can be used to cure the disease.

And so, as the symptoms persisted, I had physical exams done, along with blood work and x-rays … and, as the results filtered in, I was given muscle relaxants and opioid pain killers. In other words, my due diligence didn't result in a specific diagnosis, so it was the standard doctor's orders: "Take these pills, and if it still hurts in the morning, call me."

That was my first mistake: thinking I could outsmart, outplay, the stalking Coyote named Cancer by relying on conventional medicine. What's even worse is that I will find myself repeating this same mistake time and again … trying to outsmart the Coyote and then letting conventional medicine have its way with me.

III

Flummoxed: I am tired. The rocking of the ambulance is mesmerizing. Maybe I am dreaming. In this state of mind I am forced to accept the realization that being outsmarted and outwitted by Coyote has just now, overnight, flipped my world. I have been flummoxed by Coyote Cancer. My new world, as I'm seeing it in dream-state from the innards of an ambulance, is bewildering, baffling, and befuddling. It is unlikely that anything will ever be the same for me again.

A horn honks. Is it ours? Or some pissed-off driver, angry that someone, some *Other*, strapped to a stretcher, is getting the right of way? Either way, I am alert and focused, tensed against the possibility of a wreck. In this context of being refocused I realize: This is not the first time I've ever been flummoxed.

I've been flummoxed lots of times. Most people have. We've all had our life's crises that we've been able to work through one way or another. But when you live large, as I have long tried to do, you are constantly putting yourself into new and different living-on-the-edge situations; situations where flummoxing is one of the common outcomes.

I've been flummoxed, for example, when faced with yet another new job description, a description of tasks I have no idea how I'll ever get accomplished. Most people have had a few of these, but I've had more than my share: One HR person, during my interview and while he was thrumming his fingers over my resume, looked up and said, rather caustically: "This is the most restless resume I've ever seen."

Well, I didn't get *that* job. But over the years, I've had many new jobs -- and each has carried with it the likelihood of being flummoxed, at least at first.

For example: My first time running onto the gridiron at Iowa State's West Stadium (now converted into a parking lot for an apartment complex), fans cheering, me a starting end for the first time, my "job" at the time. Then another: My first time in the cockpit of a United 737. "Hello Captain, I'm Randy Kidd. I'll be your second officer today." Me, in both of those start-up instances, in the grips of being flummoxed ... but both of them merely the beginnings of what eventually became the routine grind of work.

On the other side of the sword, however, there was that time, sweaty after our freshman game against Nebraska, sitting next to my locker, nursing an ankle they had taped and X-rayed because they thought it was broken, when Coach came up and said: "Kidd, we have some bad news. Your father has just been killed in a plane crash. We have it set up so you can fly home for the funeral, then fly back here afterwards. Tom will take you to the airport as soon as you get dressed. Your mother knows you're coming and will pick you up at the airport. Sorry I had to tell you this."

With that said, Coach turned and quickly walked away.

Now that one was a life changing flummoxing, told in the way of warrior-speak, told by an old-school coach who expected his players to be hard-nosed, tough as nails, and full of grit. It was a flummoxing that I'm not sure I've fully recovered from to this day, more than six decades later.

IV

Last Words: Flummoxing can be a temporary "it is what it is" type of thing or it can be one that eats at you for a lifetime. Or you can be flummoxed with joy.

My absolute favorite times being flummoxed were those three times when the nurse handed me one of our newborn daughters and let me cradle her. Then, when that daughter looked up, peered directly into my eyes. When our eyes met, spirit to soul -- flummoxed by it all, I knew back then that those moments would turn my life totally around.

Some flummoxings can make your eyes water; can put a wobble into your knees; can be moments of pure joy.

Chapter 3 Interlude: Maybe; Maybe Not

I

Introduction: Thinking about flummoxings, I remember my favorite Zen story about being non-judgemental or at least withholding judgment until the full story has played out. The following is one version of that story.

II

Maybe; Maybe Not: Once upon a time there was an old farmer who had worked his crops for many years and finally had saved up enough to buy the horse he had always wanted. One day his horse ran away. Upon hearing the news, his neighbors came to visit. "Such bad luck," they said sympathetically.

"Maybe; maybe not. Too soon to tell," the farmer replied.

The next morning the horse returned, bringing with it three other wild horses. "How wonderful," the neighbors exclaimed.

"Maybe; maybe not. Too soon to tell," replied the old man.

The following day, his son tried to ride one of the untamed horses, was thrown, and broke his leg. The neighbors again came to offer their sympathy on his misfortune.

"Maybe; maybe not," answered the farmer.

The day after, military officials came to the village to draft young men into the army. Seeing that the son's leg was broken, they passed him by. The neighbors congratulated the farmer on how well things had turned out.

"Maybe," said the farmer.

III

My Maybe Stories: The stories of my life, like most of our life stories, have been reflections of the above Zen tale.

Sometimes the story is all sunshine and roses. The life stories of my three daughters and all their accomplishments, for example; the still-brewing stories of their children (our grandchildren); and the just beginning stories of our great-grandchildren. These stories couldn't be brighter; couldn't have a fresher fragrance.

Other times our life story starts out all foggy and fetid, and the sunshine never breaks through; the stench may linger for a lifetime. The far-too-early-death of my dad, for example. So many joyous moments we could have shared; so much dad-to-son-to-dad wisdom that could have been passed back and forth.

Or being diagnosed with terminal cancer – the beginning of the definitive end.

Most times though, the storyline passes through cycles of unbridled joy through dismal disappointment back to a happy ending to that story … and then repeat with a new story line. Most of the time our stories vacillate from good to bad and back again. Back and forth; back and forth.

At age 18 Sue and I got married in a fever, hotter than two pepper sprouts. You might think there would be no way but down from this hormonally-driven high. But, even given some of those troublesome instances where the peppers of life scorched our tonsils, we've always seemed able to keep our love for each other – if not always at fever pitch, at least in the temperate zone.

IV

Last Words: You never know which direction the story line will take you. I will find, as the years go on after my cancer diagnosis – one of the darkest moments of my life – that at the end of the fog, this *dis*-ease may well have created some of the best moments of my lifetime. Maybe blessings in disguise.

Pre Op

I

Through These Portals: Traffic is heavier now; we are nearing the city. The ambulance rocks right and left as we weave in and out of traffic; I am jolted wide awake as we brake and accelerate. My mind is still pondering The Big Question: "How the hell did I get here?" And now that I am getting close to where they will unload me, The Really Big Question (RBQ): "Where do I go from here?"

We drive under the archway that acts as final portal into one of Western Medicine's citadels: K.U. Med. They unload me through the mouth of Jonah's whale … or is it the gaping maw of a snake? It's been a tight fit in there, hot and humid. I take one big gulp of fresh air, look back to the doors into the ambulance, realize it is not a whale nor a snake after all. For some reason – a thinking well beyond me, far beyond normal or rational thoughts – the image of a snake or whale transforms into womb, and to emergence, and to rebirth.

I am released from my restraints and helped into a wheelchair.

I don't think I've ever been in a wheelchair before, but this one signifies one more loss of power – the power of my legs. In football you learn that the best way to take the power from an opponent is to cut his legs out from under him. "Stay low! Hit low!" our coaches kept yelling at us.

Our trainer, Brick Bickerstaff, would never let us fool around with crutches. "That's bad luck guys," he'd say. "Start fooling around with those damned things and before you know it, you'll need them just to walk across the room."

I sit in my wheelchair, waiting in a long hallway, dank and sterilized of all color and feel – waiting for someone to appear and wheel me away, someone they have promised will appear soon.

Sue finally arrives, walking down the long hallway. She shakes her head, says: "Well, I finally got you admitted, after they made absolutely certain our insurance was good and up to date." She continues, "They don't have any room on the pre-op floor, so they'll have to put you on the bariatric floor for now, whatever that is. Supposedly someone will be here shortly to wheel you up there."

I say, "Fat guy floor." She looks at me and asks, "Huh?" I say, "Bariatric. Fat guy." She nods, says, "Maybe they can whack off some of that innertube."

Another long delay, sitting there, silently. This process of getting checked into the hospital is taking forever. Don't they know I have only so long to live? Plus, I have to pee.

II

Pre-Op Whirlwind: After an interminably long wait at the entry portal to the hospital, a guy comes, makes me repeat my name, date of birth, and if I feel safe at home...for the umpteenth-plus-one time. Then he wheels me into the elevator and up to my cell.

I am met by a gaggle of bubbly-friendly nurses who do their best to make sure Sue and I are made comfortable while I am being interrogated by a steady stream of one group after another: Doctors who make sure to announce their title – admitting physician, pre-op doctor, anesthesiologist, radiologist, OR assistant doctors, post-op doctors, on and on ad infinitum, ad absurdum. They are followed by another stream of bodies, this time it's interns, nurses, sorority pledges, and whoever else happens to be walking down the hall at the time.

They help me into the hospital dress that leaves your ass open for the world to see, hook me up to a battalion of machines, insert an IV into each arm, force a catheter up my penis. They check to see that all systems are "go": steady electronic beeping of machines (that has already become an irritatingly rhythmic echo), IV fluids flowing in, bloody urine leaking into a collection bag. They ask me if I am comfortable. I lie: "Yes," I say. "Thank you."

III

My Surgeon: In a surprise move, my surgeon appears. She is a pleasingly plump lady with a pleasant personality who carries her light Welsh accent with a hint of pride. She says, "We will operate Saturday morning, the earliest time I can get a surgery room reserved. We'll let you know what time that will be. You will have another MRI sometime this evening, whenever we can get it scheduled – for some reason LMH can't figure out how to Fax their copy over." With that said, she turns and leaves the room.

There are three things I take away from her visit:

First: The oops about the MRI getting stuck in the local pony express mail. Is this an omen for things to come? I can only hope they are taking good care of the pony.

Second: The quickness of the surgeon's visit, the rapid set-up for surgery, and on a Saturday no less – all this makes it look like this is, after all, a STAT condition, one that she thinks warrants a rapid response. One more reason for me to be worried.

And finally: It's a "she", my surgeon, that is. And to me that's good news; couldn't be better. I really don't want some testosterone-fueled, positive-aggressive, ham-handed guy hacking away at me – especially in an area that requires the soft and focused and meticulous and competent touch of a female hand... so that I might be able to walk again.

So, my surgeon-to-be is a member of the female gender, eh. Thank the gods!

IV

Pre-Op: And so, I'll wait for the morrow – with some trepidation and some positive thoughts. I settle in. Sue leaves, says she'll be back later. The nurses show me how to use the TV, tell me I am not to walk without their help. I am tired. After about 15 minutes of afternoon TV, I am also bored.

I drift off. For what must be a good 5 or 6 minutes. I feel a nudge. "James, sorry to wake you, but we need to check your blood pressure, your IV, and have you answer some questions. Can you tell me your full name and date of birth? Do you feel safe at home?" And on. This is a routine I will undergo, every hour on the hour, throughout the rest of the afternoon and night. On one of those visits the nurse informs me that my surgery is scheduled for 6 AM tomorrow. Six in the morning!? Well, I'll be damned! Ah well.

A question keeps brooding, has my mind working full-bore, has me stirring in my dreams: I wonder if I'd be better off in the hands of one of those natural healers – an acupuncturist, say, or an herbalist, a Native American Shaman/root doctor, or a homeopath. I'm familiar with all these medicines because I've used them in my veterinary holistic practice...or I have seen them used in other venues.

As time creeps along, listening to the steady beeping of machines, I can't help but wonder what it would feel like having a shaman shake his rattle over me; can't help wonder where the acupuncturist would place the needles, where I would place the needles were I my own patient. I try to remember which herbs I might use, try to figure which homeopathic remedy might work.

V

Last Words: At the same time I'm thinking thoughts of alternatives, I realize this situation with a tumor affecting critical areas of my body is exactly what Western Medicine is made for, exactly what it is best at treating. Realizing all this, I am still not totally comforted, but I can breathe a tad bit easier.

I take a deep breath, my mind moves into a reverie state and begins to daydream of days long ago past.

Chapter 4 Interlude: Cold-Cocked

I

Cold-cocked: My daydream takes me back to Autumn, early 1960s, back in the day. Back when the stud within me would run short crossing routes and dare the sissy-assed linebackers to try to hit me hard enough to jar the ball loose. Back when that tactic backfired on me. Back when I got head-hit by a linebacker a good 100 pounds my superior. Cold-cocked.

That's the day when I gave our trainer, Brick Bickerstaff, what was to become one of his favorite stories to tell.

Typically, Brick's story would begin as we were waiting in the lobby for the bus to take us to the game day locker room. Brick would round up some of his cronies from the trainer bunch or from his war days, and then he'd call me over to be part of his show-and-tell that would go something like this:

"I knew when Kidd hit the ground and stayed down, he'd been hit pretty hard. He's one of our tough-guy players. So, I trotted over, and I got on top of him, straddled his chest so I could check to make sure he was breathing."

"Good thing I'd hurried, too," he'd continue, "cause when he started to come to, he came out of it running. Squirming. Legs in the air, pumping the sky like he was running a long route on the bottom side of clouds. About all I could do to hold him down, me sitting on his chest."

"I had him held down pretty good, though," Brick continues with a chuckle, "and he kept asking, 'Where the fuck am I? Where the fuck am I? Where the fuck am I?' All the time, running in the air. Funniest thing I've ever seen." By now, Brick would be laughing out loud.

"You remember that, Kidd?" he'd ask me, and both of us already knew the answer. "Nope."

"You even remember what it was hit you?"

"Not a clue, Brick, not a clue. Felt like a cement truck, though, going about 80." And everyone gathered there would have a good laugh.

II

Memories: It's true: I don't remember a thing about that cold-cocking which happened during a Wednesday evening practice. Nor do I remember getting home after practice and not recognizing that strange woman, sitting there talking to me – that woman who I later figured out was in fact Sue, the woman I'd been married to for more than two years.

Interestingly I also don't remember anything about most of the day before I took the hit – there are hours before I got cold-cocked that I have no recollection of. Totally lost and gone hours.

Teammates tell me I acted strange during our after-practice team meetings and even walked into the wrong meeting room – until someone led me back into the hall and pointed me toward the room I was supposed to be in.

The first thing I remember after taking that hit was waking up at about 3:00 am, sitting up in bed, and, for the first few minutes, wondering where the fuck I was…until, after several more minutes sitting there, I finally figured it out. I'll be damned. I'm home.

I can remember that Sue took me to the hospital the next morning where Doc H, our team physician, put a stethoscope to my chest for a few seconds, told me to breathe in deep … and cleared me to practice. I remember playing my usual 35-45 minutes in the game that next Saturday, although I don't think I had one of my better games.

And, Sue continues to remind me how scared she was that night when I didn't recognize her.

I also remember the game a year later when my mom flew out from Ohio to see me play, my only college game she would get to see. I remember that Sue, after the game, could tell that I didn't recognize my own mother – I'd been dinged again. She quickly pulled me aside and pointed toward my mom, said: "Your Mother," and led me to her side.

My dad, by the way, never got to see me play college ball; he was killed during my freshman year at ISU when the National Guard plane he was piloting went down. So, sadly, he never got to see the hard-nosed, tough-assed ball player he had helped me become.

III

Part of the Game: Getting *cold-cocked*, having your *bell rung*, getting *head-dinged* were all a part of the game back in the day; in my case, a relatively frequent part of the game.

There were dozens of times, dating back to high school, when I'd had my bell rung. Times when I wouldn't know where I was for a few minutes -- or, in some cases, for a few hours. Dozens of other times when I'd just been head-dinged and one side or the other of my body would go completely dead, totally numbed out. Anesthetic without having to pay the anesthesiologist.

One can only wonder what amount of residual brain ad-dling I have today as the result of all the dinging, bell-ringing, cold-cocking … or whatever you want to call it. It's all a part of what I carry with me to this day, the benefit package of having played college football.

IV

Last Words: I do remember that there was one positive to having your bell rung: The ringing inside your head was so loud you couldn't hear the coaches yelling at you – a real blessing. About all you could do when you saw the froth at the corner of their mouth was to head-bobble, look the screamer in the eye, nod, and say "yes sir."

The O.R. and The Post OP ICU

I

The O.R. I am jolted awake: "James, it's time for your surgery. Can you tell me your whole name and date of birth and if you feel safe at home?" The nurses help me out of my hospital bed onto the wheeled gurney. One asks: "James, do you want another blanket to help cover you up?" I say, "Nah. Nothing to see there anyway." I'm thinking: if I die during surgery, the size of my penis won't make any difference.

She laughs, says, "You wouldn't believe some guys. They'll let it flop out so anyone along the hallway can see it, laying there as if they're proud as they can be of it. I always want to say: 'No need for that here, buster. You're not impressing any of us." Some banter to pass the time as I'm being wheeled down the hall, without being able to show off my true prowess ... one last time before I die.

We enter the OR – so bright you need to squint to see anything at all. When my eyes have adjusted, I see that everyone is masked and gowned up, only their eyes showing. Through the lights, a voice: "Hi James, I am Doctor XYZ, your anesthesiologist." There is a moment of fright, realizing that anesthesia can be a lethal intervention.[1] Doctor XYZ continues: "You have been given a pre-anesthetic, and ... now ... we ... will ...."

---

1 Anesthesia has always carried with it the threat of death – although that threat in today's operating room (OR) is minimal. Anesthesia related mortality has fallen from 64 per 100,000 patients in the 1940's to less than one per 100,000 patients at present (somewhere between 0.4 to 0.8 per 100,000 depending on the study being used). This rate applies to patients without systemic disease; mortality is higher among patients with severe accompanying illnesses and in older patients.

Overall, mortality within the first postoperative year is still disturbingly high. One study found that after an operation under general anesthesia, 5.5% of all patients died within one year, and in patients older than 65 years the proportion rose to 10.3%. (Monk TG, et al. Anesthetic management and one-year mortality after noncardiac surgery. Anesth Analg 2005; 100:4-10 [PubMed] [Google Scholar])

He fades into the glare; then, the fog, coming in on little coyote paws, slowly eats his face. I try to follow other faces as they move slowly about the room with unhurried and practiced competence. Their eyes, sunken into flesh between the surgery mask and cap, turn to yellow, glowing. Those eyes move about, pacing, focused on their prey. I try to keep my eyes on the circling, tensing for their inevitable attack. Fur grows around masks. Ears elongate, become pointed.

Noses and jaws lengthen, become muzzles, an occasional ivory glint of long canine teeth. Is that me, floating above the lights close to the ceiling? Me in a flowing white gown, ghostlike. An apparition. These are the last images I remember … before the portal into my cranial vault opens, let's the fog creep in, blanketing my brain.

II

Post Op I.C.U.: Is "waking up" the proper term for what happens when you *come out* of being *put under* general anesthesia?

My waking up is slow and tentative – at first I am able to convince myself that I might still be alive; the next instant I am absolutely certain I am no longer of this world. I know not where I am nor who I am … or even if I still am.

My mind is a fuzz-ball; that damnably infernal sun-bright of artificial light overhead clouds my vision and my world is slowly spinning – first spinning, then gently swaying back and forth with the wind in the treetops. The trees: the fluttering of leaf against leaf; I think they are the leaves of cottonwoods. I am now, hunkered down, nested, in the spinning wind of treetops.

But really, where the hell am I? Hell? Or somewhere else that only looks, smells and feels like hell – a living hell of the glaring flame of bright lights, and the incessant click, click, clicking … mingled with the unnerving background hum and thrum of monitoring-machinery at work. Machinery I am hooked up to and that monitors who I am now – and then regurgitates occult numbers that some highly-trained being (and hopefully an alive and well – and awake – being) will try to interpret.

My vision clears just enough to see those long-snouted, furred forms with fangs that I remember from just before I *went under* the anesthetic. They move, ghost-like, around the room, circling me. I test to see if flight is still an option, but I am trapped by straps coiled around my body, more straps holding my legs in the web of a blanketed cocoon. I can't feel my legs, let alone move them. Fight is my next option … but I have no juice left, not an ounce of fight left in me. *J'ai perdu mon saut … I have lost my oomph!*

So, freeze it is. Perhaps if I freeze, none of those forms will notice me lying here, easy prey.

I hear the forms murmuring quietly to each other, although I cannot tell what they are saying … or even what language they are using. Gradually, very slowly, the forms are transformed into eerie shadows on the wall, still ghost-like, growing long and tall like tree trunks, then, as they move about, shrinking into small shadow-puddles on the floor. They move with the grace of smoke, smoke carried by the circling of winds at the leading edge of a storm. I am trapped in Plato's cave, unable to create a rational thought, unable to escape.

After a while, I can refocus, my eyes able to see what is closer to my bed. The shadows become moving figures, almost humanoid in appearance. They lose fangs, then fur, and finally snouts that I now see are surgical masks hooked over noses and protruding from faces. Real human faces.

I remember being told that my face would be swollen after surgery since I would have been lying face down with my face in a supporting donut for several hours. And yes, my face feels like a bloated tick, fat with blood, my blood. I try to talk. I slur a few words that even I can't decipher.

Gradually, ever so slowly, I feel a watery ebb and flow of heat and energy that begins to revitalize my body. It is a pulsing, emanating from that collapsed coil of energetics and muscle that lives just in front of where my tumor had been. It is the vibrant pulse of my heart, working ever outward in concentric circles.

The swelling around my eyes must be receding because I can focus a little better now. I try to speak again, and this time I almost recognize the words, coming from deep within a cave … although I still can't understand what I'm saying. I doze: in and out of sleep, in and out of consciousness and awareness, in and out of coherence.

During one of my more coherent moments, I recognize Sue sitting nearby, and have the good sense to say something like: "Oh, thank God. I must be in heaven. I see an angel right here next to me." Sue does not look impressed.

Sue tells me later that I was very chatty during all the time I was in the ICU. Says the nurses were actually very kind and didn't tell me to shut the fuck up. Not even once. What's more, I don't think I said: "Where the fuck am I?" even once during my chattiness, but I cannot be certain about that.

I will later learn how the miracle of surgery extracted my tumor. Using a surgical bone saw my miracle-worker female surgeon sliced off the tops of three thoracic vertebrae – the entire top of thoracic-2 (T-2) along with the distal end of T-1 and the proximal end of T-3. (In horses, this is where the withers are.)[2]

I will carry with me the hole in the withers of my spine ... until the day I die. But, thanks to my miracle-worker surgeon I no longer have that nasty tumor that was pushing my spinal cord out of its canal.

III

Last Words: I have just been put through (and thus far have survived) one simple thread of life's essence – an essence that weaves its spun-fibers together to create the very fabric of consciousness. My journey began with the basic level of awake and aware consciousness, proceeded via general anesthesia into unconsciousness, and is now gradually coming back to consciousness ... with several grey zones in between.

This is not my first rodeo for this type of journey. I've been put under anesthesia for several previous operations. I survived all those, and now it looks like I will survive this one also.

The question now is, as it is with all such journeys: What, if anything, did I leave behind on this journey? Shamans suggest

---

2 Today's surgical bone saws are not what the Sawbones docs of yore used, applying human-hand power to scrape the saw across bone and tissue. Today's models are typically power-driven and reciprocating, oscillating at something like 32,000 oscillations per minute (or @540 per second) ... which is about 8 times faster than a hummingbird's wing beat. The cut is much more accurate ... but the saws cut damnably fast. So, I had to rely on the skilled hands of my OR doctor to leave my spinal cord intact.

that I have likely left behind a part of my soul, and one of the ways shamans heal is to return one's soul to its rightful place.

Chapter 5 Interlude: Coyote

I

Coyote Visits: Between nurse visits I drift in and out of dream state, and Coyote keeps appearing in my dreams – not a big surprise since Coyote has been given to me as one of my power animals. What is a surprise is that he can so easily shape shift into hospital garb…and that he seems to always be walking along in a thin fog while visiting.

II

Wise Coyote: Following are some of Coyote's gifts while visiting – the pearls of his wisdom, and the ways he uses to apply that wisdom:

Coyote is the consummate trickster, always playing with your mind, flipping situations so he can get away with his antics. He is a master at shape shifting or disguising himself, so you never know who he really is; acting silly so you don't notice the chicken in his mouth he has just stolen from you. Coyote always looks out for himself, as I like to say: "living large" – satisfying his ravenous appetites, nutritional, emotional, and sexual.

In my pre- and post-op daydreams Coyote is more the ghost dog he is often described as; his image appears, then disappears into the woods as a specter. You think you see him; then you don't. You are never sure.

As I am forced more and more to deal with the reality of my cancer, I will learn that cancer in general exhibits almost all the traits ascribed to Coyote, the Trickster Exemplar: a) as a disease, cancer is fundamentally a deceiver and trick-player – clinical signs leading to diagnosis are often ambiguous and anomalous; b) cancer is both a shape shifter and a master of disguise; c) cancer cells often invert situations – they are often the epitome of what a healthy, voraciously growing and reproducing cell culture might look like…if it hadn't gone crazy out of control.

In addition: d) cancers may have a sacred and lewd brico-
leur – this is especially true in my case where the cancerous cells
originated in a sexual organ (prostate) and initially grew in the
area of my sacrum (from the Greek for "sacred bone") and are
now – wreaking their havoc by dissolving the bones along my
spine, from stem (upper back) to stern (hips).

And finally, there is the possibility that a particular cancer
might be the e) messenger and imitator of the gods. Who knows
about this one, but in my case, I'm willing to listen for any message from the gods.

III

Last Words: Since I'll be dealing with a trickster-of-a-disease,
an exemplar of trickster personified, it will behoove me to learn
all I can about trickster ways from my new partner, Coyote/Can-
cer. Thus, Coyote will, of necessity, become my tutor in Nature –
teaching me the natural ways of cancer…so I can deal with them
in my own trickster fashion.

With those thoughts, I drift into another dream where Coyote appears. Is that a strand of woven yarn he holds? A ruler?
A pair of scissors? Am I sitting at a student's desk in the middle
of the oak grove?

I have some early-on questions I intend to ask Coyote Tutor,
such as: Will I be able to listen hard enough and deep enough
for the message within the coyote howl? Will I have the courage
to walk with Nature, to listen to the teachings She has to offer,
and to learn from them? And finally, will I have enough respect
for Nature's Coyotes…to let them show me how I should come
to terms with my disease. Naturally.

Only time will tell.

Recovery

I

Survival Skills: Strange things come to mind when you are regaining your mind after having it absorbed into the brew from the anesthesiologist's cauldron. Some folks claim to see angels when coming out of anesthesia; others speak of dreaming about their life's greatest accomplishments. Apparently, I remember those places of life where I've gone through the worst … and survived. My survival moments.

I'm feeling pretty damned proud of myself. I've been *cold-cocked* on the gridiron, and I've gone under general anesthesia ... and it looks like I'll survive both. Two different inputs with the same output: you lose consciousness for a period of time, and then somehow, as if by magic, you are returned back to the "normal" world. I even know, or think I know, where the fuck I am.

The one thing I don't yet know is whether I'll ever be able to use my legs. Once again, I test to see if I can raise them, pump them into the air while shouting: Where the fuck am I? Then I remember that I am cocooned into blankets, and straps hold me to the gurney. Something more to worry about while the nurses hover around, making sure I don't croak on their watch.

They observe intently as I move into more and more awakeness, gradually becoming more and more aware of where and who I am. As I've said, this is not my first rodeo for this type of journey – a journey that transports you from consciousness to unconsciousness and back to consciousness again.

It is, however, my first rodeo where I am being asked to ride the roughstock called cancer. I will discover later that this particular ride is ultimately not tame-able. The genetic bloodline of my cancer beast will eventually find a way to buck me off. At least that's what the oncologists will tell me – maybe next year's silver-bullet cancer cure will work; but for now, according to the experts, nothing has worked for more than a few extra months. (In cowboy time, that might give me a six or seven second ride … but not the full eight.)

Today's drugs may work for those few months and let you stay with the ride. Then the bronc, without warning, turns rank to the feel of the flank strap, drops suddenly, and before gravity lets you resettle onto his back, heaves himself back into thin air … leaving you without rein or seat. Trying to ride cancer's Stage 4 prostate mount, you will ultimately end up in a heap of fractured bones. In the dust. Dust to dust.

I will also find out, from painful experience, that some of the drugs they use to "extend" your life's ride will be so befogging of body/mind/soul as to render you nearly unconscious and almost totally beholden to the beast.

I will learn, after many falls off the cancer bronc, that there are a few natural ways of staying the ride. I will learn that staying in motion – riding along with the bronc's bucking and heaving – is more effective than trying to overpower it by tugging on its reins. I will learn that nature has many ways to show us how to sit a horse, even that rank horse angry enough to buck us off and kick us in the head on our way down.

Finally, I will learn that, if you allow it to happen, a nasty bronc – even a bucking horse with the power of life and death over you … can enhance focus, creativity, and love. In other words, I will learn that even terminal cancer can be one of life's greatest blessings. But those teachings will come later. Much later.

Right now I am being wheeled out of the ICU toward somewhere else. The somewhere else turns out to be the Fat Guy ward.

II

Doing Time: The post-op nurses have given me my sentence as I am being wheeled out through the portals of the ICU into the halls leading to the bariatric floor: several days, maybe a week or so, they say. I am wheeled into my cell, unstrapped, and rolled over onto one of those beds with steel fencing on both sides. I check for razor wire atop the fencing. None. Perhaps there is hope for escape yet. I begin to lay out my plans.

I am to reside in a solitary cell in the obesity ward of the hospital. There will be an empty bed next to me for the duration of my stay. I am told that I am on the fat guy floor of the hospital because the ER and Post Op beds are full, it being a holiday and all.

Both of my arms are hooked into IVs; incoming stuff: fluids and who knows what else. I am catheterized, outgoing stuff: bloody urine. A helpful aide shows me, once again, how to use the TV, how to push the red call-button when I need anything. I am told, once again, I am not to try to walk anywhere, anytime, without assistance. Everyone is friendly, quietly efficient, and full of compassion. The stench of sterilized hospital is nearly overwhelming.

I check to see where the exits are positioned – a habit I learned while sitting on barstools in those seedy bars I used to frequent. Best to have an exit plan already in place.

Sue asks if I'm OK, says she has some things to do, and she'll be back as soon as she's done. I stare at the walls, eventually fall asleep, and as soon as I'm asleep, a nurse comes in, wakes me up, asks what I want for dinner. I order from the hospital menu and turn on the TV.

It's a routine I will become accustomed to over the next few days. I stare at barren white walls. Eat, sleep, and be awakened by a nurse for prodding, puncturing and questions about how I feel. Am I safe at home, can I repeat my full name and birthdate? Stare at wall. Try to watch TV. Fall asleep. Repeat.

Who knew commercial TV could be so interesting in its very banality? You can just see very creative twelve-year-old minds, working in their Platonic cave-like cubicles, giggling madly when their best efforts produce exactly what their mass audience craves: the ultimate of the trite.

I am held rapt by the offerings: serial killers are profiled, drug dealers tell their stories. (Did you know that a hotbed for drug dealing is Utah? Apparently devout Mormons have found bliss in drugs.). There are 5,255 ways (at least) to create a reality show where folks yell at each other in unreal ways. Singing, dancing, cooking have all become spectator sports – their competitions much followed by the perpetually bored and lonely. And much, much more. So much more blah.

After TV, it gets no better in the bariatric ward. Who knew that being unable to take care of yourself could be so demeaning – to both self and to those who tend to your personal care. I find myself feeling sorry for the young male newbie-nurse who is steadying me in the shower as he soaps up my ass. I vow to get to self sufficiency as quickly as possible.

III

Plan Ahead: I make my first promise to self and others who will be around me – especially Sue: I will not let myself become a burden. It is the first in many long lists I will devise for myself: lists of action plans to include my personal credo, or a manifesto for dealing with cancer, or my list of tenets or principles by which I will live this next, cancer-ridden life of mine … or simply a list of "Some of the Stuff I Hope to Live My Life By Today" – my To Do Today List.

I will discover only much later on that the combo of cancer and chemo drug side effects will, on many days, make it almost impossible to achieve anything beyond a long daily nap. I call these my "Crash Days" – days when Sue gets to watch me hibernating, curled up in my hibernaculum … er, on the couch. Most other days I will be operating at half speed … or less.

And so, until wishes become horses, living a life around pre-formed goals and objectives will not be in my immediate future.

Furthermore, it will turn out that the "Do Not A Burden Be" promise will be the one most difficult to achieve. I had not counted on the toll of the dark cloud of death constantly at the doorstep being as potent as it is -- reminding, always reminding you and yours of your encrypted future. Always the reminder that you ain't quite right … and you never will be.

And so, in addition to not being a burden, I eventually pare down my daily To-Do list to include just four legs: 1) Take a daily walk … because *"motion is lotion."* 2) make that a walk in Nature … whenever weather allows. 3) stay in touch with family and keep them up to date in my progress (or lack of progress). 4) take a stab at trying to stay creative via writing.

The tail that walks this four-legged dog is my basic life theme: **"Reuniting the Human Spirit with the Soul of Nature."**

IV

Last Words: Back to the hum and humdrum of the hospital. I try to read, but can't concentrate. Sue and I talk, first about general stuff, then as time wears on, about the stuff that really matters – Life. How lucky we've been to have lived the life we have. How blessed we are to have the children and family we have. How much I appreciate all these things. How much I love where we've been, what we've done, even the where and what of how we find ourselves today, less than a week after my cancer diagnosis. How much I appreciate this time we have together to talk about all these things.

Eventually we will get around to talking about death. Death on my doorstep, the guy with the scythe patiently waiting there for me.

Time will become a very special aspect of my type of cancer: notably, Stage 4 prostate cancer gives the average patient 3 to 5 years to live – with only a paltry few souls still alive after that fifth year. No matter the therapy (or lack of therapy), the guy with the scythe will almost certainly come a'knockin' sometime during those five years.

Three to five. Danged, that's short. But … with some luck, it will give us – Sue and I and our family – a few years of time together. And it will give us that time knowing this is a terminal disease.

In other words, unlike many other cancers (and anything else that causes sudden death, such as lightning strike, car or airplane accident, or being bitten by a bushmaster snake), you've been given some time, Buster. And no matter how hard you look for a cure, there ain't one out there – at least not yet. Make the absolute best use of the time you're given Big Guy!

Physical Therapy: Meanwhile, within all the humdrum of being institutionalized in sterility, in the bariatrics ward, a moment of great joy actually manages to come along one afternoon. A PT (physical therapist) is assigned to see if she can get me up and about, back to walking, possibly walking like a normal guy would.

Chapter 6 Interlude: Coyote in PT Clothes

I

My PT (Physical Therapist): We meet. When I struggle my way to the stand-up position, we are nearly eye-level. She is at least two inches taller. Lithe as a mountain lion, obviously an athlete.

I've grown accustomed to this type of tall athleticism. Sue and I have had, over the past few years, three young ladies (our granddaughters) who played collegiate volleyball, and one son-in-law and one grandson who both played collegiate basketball, and one grandson-in-law who pitched collegiately. We've thus been blessed with having met and befriended many lithe and competent tall-folks who were often taller (and more athletic) than I ever was.

I ask my PT person, "So where did you play ball?"

"KU. Volleyball," she says. "Only two years though. Had to quit when I got into the PT program."

"What was your vertical?"

"Low 30s," she says, "Maybe mid 30s," with a smile.

"How close could you come to that today?" I ask. She laughs.

II

In Action: My PT and I are walking the corridors of the hospital; I am using one of the hospital's two-wheeled, two-pegged walkers. Someone found this walker hidden away in a long-ago-forgotten closet. The walker I'd been using before physical therapy was a bariatric one – handles wide enough apart to fit a 600-pound silver-back gorilla. This one I fit into without extending my arms straight out.

I walk along, with the PT person behind, holding onto the belt around my fat guy middle so I won't fall. When I feel her let go of her death grip, I'm thinking proud, thinking I'm doing pretty good, so I say something like: "They tell me my being pigeon-toed was one reason I'm such a good sprinter." Then I ask, expecting the appropriate ego-massage: "How's my gait look to you?"

She answers, and I'm guessing she says this straight-faced: "Well, you still have some bilateral toe-drag, and you tend to walk with a scissor gait. That means you're sashaying from one side to another, kinda prissy like. All this is pretty normal after spinal surgery. You may eventually get back to a more normal gait … or you may never get there."

So much for ego boosting. I'm thinking: I damned well better get rid of that prissy look. Somehow.

III

Our Hallway! And so, it's back to round and round in hospital hallway circles. I think she is as bored as I am. We round a corner, and she pulls me aside. "See that bunch of white jackets down there, all hunched over their damned portable computer units. That's a flock of intern docs. They always think they own the hallways. I want you to walk straight through them, just like it's your hallway. Like you own it."

I nod. Get my grit-look on. Hunker down low into the walker. Set my pace as fast as I can without falling down – which is still creep-speed. Head for the middle of the group. Don't say a word until I'm about three or four paces away.

Then, as they finally look up and scatter to the sides of the hallway like a covey of feeding quail when the coyote pounces, I offer: "Oh, sorry there. Excuse me. Pardon me." And I keep moving on.

We get to the end of the hall, turn the corner where I have to pause, exhausted. Try to catch my breath. My PT hi-fives, says with a huge grin, "Good job. You're good to go." And she signs me off, able to go home.

IV

Last Words: My coyote-pounce on the hallway interns gave me a taste of coyote credibility once again. Enough cred, anyway, that I get sent home a few days earlier than expected. Me and My Coyote, doing our dance one more time.

PART TWO: Reclaiming Life

Home Again

Home Again, Home Again, Jiggety-Jig: They wheel-chair me to the backdoor of the hospital where Sue is to pick me up. I am told that the walker I have been given to take home is a gift from the government – read that "Medicare" -- but that it is the only one I will get for three years. "Make it last" is the obvious message.

Sue and I are silent for the ride from KU Med to Lawrence – too much to think about. We are not really returning to our final home. We have been living in an apartment, temporary quarters while the construction company, Real Estate Equities (REE), finishes building the old-folks cooperative-living residence we have signed up for. When completed, it will be a 50-unit complex referred to as The Village Co-op of Lawrence (VCL), or more simply to most of us old folks who will live there, "the Village", or even more simply "the Coop."

The Village is already six months behind on their supposed-to-be schedule, the timeline we were given when we bought into the project. It's a six-month lag that will serve as a major indicator and the very beginnings of the massive list of frustrations yet to come – more than five years filled with those frustrations. This disease that some people insist on referring to as the "construction industry" will soon become the second cancer that I will need to deal with.

And so, our "home" is not really a home; it's an apartment we are camping in until the Village Coop of Lawrence gets finished and we can move into our future (and last, or terminal) home.

There will be days of boredom, dozing off, and thinking – always thinking, cogitating about what now. Nights will be filled with trying to sleep and dreaming, always dreaming, strange dreams that seem to have no purpose or meaning.

Overall we will spend more than two years in our Camson Apartments, until we are finally able to move into our cooperative unit. (The Camson name, according to a Google search, means: affectionate, inventive, trustworthy – none of which apply to our stay there.)

While in Camson Apartments, I will undergo initial chemo-therapy, learn to walk again, attempt to learn how to think again, try to write, keep on keeping on, and do my best, under the circumstances, to reconnect with Nature. It will be a very enlightening two years, a journey of life that has, in one fell swoop, been flipped a good 180-degrees from the life I'd been living up to now.

II

Home Is Where the Poop Falls: We arrive at our "temporary" apartment, and I stumble along as Sue helps me get seated in the chair that will become my favorite (and the only one that gives my back some relief). The chair (read this *MY* chair) faces the wall that houses the TV along with a few other crunched-together pieces of furniture, some of them stacked one on top of the other.

If I want to change seats, I struggle to get up and limp along for several feet to the couch which faces a small outside deck and the lawn area where the adjacent apartment renters walk their dogs. After living there for about 18 months, I'd watched perhaps hundreds of dogs walking and pooping, and thus far, I'd seen only one person pick up his dog's poop.

It's a delightful way to spend one's days; watching dogs deposit their poop just outside your deck. I think back to the day when it was fashionable to rub a dog's nose in his deposits … to teach him a lesson. "Don't you *ever* poop on the floor again Rufus," you say in as angry a voice as you can muster, "or I'll damned sure rub your nose in it again!"

It was a training method that didn't work very well on dogs, but I'd like to try it on each and every one of the asshole dog walkers outside my window.

Watching dogs poop and the incredible offerings of daytime TV are my true delights for now. I sense the need to learn how to appreciate these small niceties of life, now set out before me … if not the need to fall in love with them. In the meantime, I am also fascinated by being able to watch how much faster the grass grows when it is fertilized with dog poop.

III

Night Flights: Nighttime viewing can be a lot less stressful. After sundown, I turn from watching pooping dogs to watching the nighttime skies. I sit in a cast iron chair on our five-by-eight-foot deck and gaze at the stars and the moon and the planes that fly by every night.

And so, I begin my night watching by trying to pick out the night flying planes overhead – easy to see with their wingtip navigational lights of red and green. Spotting the planes takes me back to the more pleasant times when I was flying cross-country night trips.

When we were flying during daytime hours and under visual conditions, we often used maps (called "Sectional Charts") which are drawn to show visual landmarks – railroads, lakes and rivers, towns and cities, football fields and stadiums, electric powerlines, the blinking lights atop towers – all of them landmarks that confirmed we were still heading in the right direction.

When we were flying under instrument conditions (and most often during night flights), we would follow designated flight paths or airline routes. These designated flight paths were defined by radio signals sent from ground-based electronic systems (VOR, Very High Frequency Omni-Directional Range, or simply *Omni* stations to us). The VOR/Omni stations provided us with what pilots know as azimuth information -- info that gives both direction and height above the ground.

In today's world I suppose all things follow the mechanized pathway that is designated by the miracle of GPS. One wonders how wild animals can find their way without all the gadgetry we humans have devised to help us.

Over the years I've come to believe everyone has their own personal pathway, their unique course to destination. And while each of us, wild and tame, has our way of being guided, we are ultimately and intricately linked to our guide ... or to those footsteps in the woods and grasslands that have formed the pathways before us.

Anyway, from my night-watching post on our apartment's deck, I try to guess where each flight is coming from and where it's headed to by watching their flight path overhead. One from the southwest flies low heading northeast – maybe from Arizona or SoCal, losing altitude to land at MCI (Kansas City's airport). Another one flying high from the east and headed about due west – possibly from STL, headed to DEN or places beyond. Another one flying low that comes to the edge of Lawrence from the south and then turns east -- likely from Wichita or Dallas/Ft. Worth and going into MCI or maybe even Lawrence Municipal. All very interesting -- if you're into watching planes.

IV

Star Gazing: From airplanes and their blinking lights I can move on into star gazing. Already I know a few stars (and our moon). But I have no want-to, no need to learn the names of all the stars, nor the arc of the planets, nor the science behind their making or what their composition is now. What I want to know is their stories, and the stories that have come to us from long ago.

It is the night watching (actually the nighttime watching, listening, ... and thinking about the stories within the stars) that ultimately gets me off my ass and back into Nature.

V

Natural Nightlights: I am entranced by the phases of the moon – each one carrying me ever nearer to the guy with the scythe. After I begin chemo, I will learn that treatments provide me with the expectation of a few months of extra lifetime – one more reason to watch moon phases.

At the start of my time-on-deck, I know a few constellations: Orion, Ursa Major and Ursa Minor. The Ursae (the Bears, Major and Minor) I know only because they point me toward the north star – a helpful hint when you are out coon hunting, lost in the woods. Or when you're looking to your North Star as a navigational guide for how to live the rest of your life.

From where I sit on my deck, I look directly down Orion's sight line. Orion is the night-sky hunter, and as I watch him aim his bow and arrow, I am reminded that – thanks to my wobblies -- I will likely never enjoy a hunt again. Nighttime hunts – always my favorites -- are even less likely.

VI

The Hunters: Orion, as night sky hunter, reminds me that we – the hunters for new lands, new beginnings, and new lives – used Orion (and the Others of the night sky) to help us navigate the vast emptiness of the ocean … as we went out to find our "other" place where we could put down new roots. Early on it was the stars we relied on, providing us with invisible pathways to our New World.

Star-lit pathways that helped guide my great great grandfather's family from an Ireland that was rapidly declining … to a land promising better times and better lives. Then too, it should be remembered that those star-lit pathways were also the same ones our ancestors leaned on to help bring with them a source of slave labor.

VII

Last Words: And thus, the stars, as guiding lights to other places, might be remembered as the shining lights of possibility … or as the evil eyes of the ogre lurking in the dark. Very seldom does Nature reveal only one pathway.

Furthermore, even before the stars were used as navigational aids, they were used as storytelling aids, as wee bits of twinkling to hitch a storyline onto. The sky is full of wonderful tales of gods and goddesses, of wars and struggles, of joy and love and hope.

Chapter 7 Interlude: Stories in the Skies

Stories in the Skies: What I find especially endearing (and entertaining) about the stories in the skies is that they are told from the perspective of the teller. That is, each tribal storyteller – and thus each separate segment of culture – has its own, very unique, story to tell ... about the stars overhead that, in reality, appear exactly the same to each of the cultures.

And isn't that a part of what Nature is really all about – providing us with enough nuance that we can make up our own stories and thus devise our own ways to live our lives.

According to the storyteller, even your own fate may be determined by your Zodiac sign – the sign in the sky you were born under. There's even some scientific evidence that points to the idea that the Zodiac month you were born under determines at least a portion of your fate.

Who's to say that the ancients didn't create permanent etchings on their brains, hunting for reality through their continual storytelling – nodal etchings that might correspond to the stars they were seeing? And who's to say that these etchings might not then form into a galaxy of connecting points of light – possibly with the central node becoming the pineal gland, the tiny, pine-cone shaped gland that modulates sleep patterns in both circadian and seasonal cycles ... much as our galaxy's sun does.

If you can suspend disbelief long enough, you could imagine a brain with anatomically fixed nodes of light that might correspond to the planets and the stars.[3] And these nodes could, with the right connections to Nature, rotate around the pineal gland in a yearly dance of neuronally rhythmic movement ... thus replicating inside what was being seen outside.

Then with the cranium as the container of the inner galaxy, it would be easy to extend the parts of the human body into other galaxies, other worlds, and other universes. One could then

3 In the 1800's a French pathologist and anatomist, Louis-Antoine Ranvier discovered nodes or gaps (Nodes of Ranvier) that occur in the myelin sheath of nerve cells. Nerve conduction in myelinated axons seems to jump from one node to the next one, resulting in faster conduction of the nerve's action potential. Perhaps these gaps/nodes were originally produced as the ancients spent so much time concentrating on the stars above and thus burning holes into the myelin sheaths of the brain's nerves – thus giving rise to anatomical reasoning for a star-filled cranium. At least that's my story ... and I'm sticking to it.

imagine the Milky Way as the storyteller's torso, complete with the white juices of digestion. And that same storyteller could imagine his legs and arms as extensions of the universe, spinning their way ever outward.

Or another, tangential story might be that, after incorporating the nightlights as an integral part of your being, you could actually see a hunter in the sky (one you named Orion); and two bears – one big one, another smaller; and seven points of light that seemed to be acting as if they were bickering sisters; or any number of other distinct images. With the night image imprinted on your mind, wouldn't you then devise a story to tell about it – a story that sang an absolute truth to what you were seeing?

Moreover, wouldn't the ancients have noticed the progression of nightlights across the skies and integrate those movements to events that happened here on earth – events such as seasonal changes that physically altered their surrounding landscape, and events such as tribal births that occurred during the seasons and created new (and often very different) kinds of personalities.

And isn't it interesting that my cancer diagnosis and tumor surgery occurred just before the appearance of the constellation Cancer, the fourth sign in the zodiac – the Cancer Constellation appearing in the form of a crab, much like how my tumor must have appeared to the surgeon.

And finally, both Sue and my Sun sign is Virgo, Latin for maiden. The maiden has a wealth of mythological lore attached to her, stories which make sense for Sue, but not for me. Until. Until, in the days to come, when I will be subjected to androgen deprivation therapy (ADT) … which will turn me into a rather buxom maiden. I await with bated breath.

Last Words: Now I know that taking life stories from the skies is scientific balderdash. And yet. And yet, isn't it also true that stories are the true essence of existence, the way we human beings actually see reality?

Well, all this being said, I am a dying man, and I don't have much time to devote to learning the stories contained in the skies. Nor to making up my own stories to tell about the skies overhead.

Owl Comes Calling

I

Owl Comes Calling: I've watched the planes go by, said my good-nights to Orion, the Bears, and the North Star, and am now lying in bed, staring at the ceiling – which is offering absolutely no info for how much longer I will live. Then, out of the night there comes a tapping, a gentle rapping from the dark of the night outside.

That's how I remember it anyway: first a tapping waking me up, then a rapping, a gentle rapping from somewhere outside our bedroom window … followed directly by the hoots and hollers of some strange creature, seemingly sitting on the rooftop right above our apartment bedroom. The sounds demand, "Who cooks for you? Who cooks for you? Who cooks for you nowww?"

Sue sits straight up, rubs her eyes, says, "What the hell?"

"Must be a Barred Owl on our rooftop," I say. "Let's go check."

We tumble out of bed, I into my pants, Sue into her robe, and we are off, stumbling down the stairway to the front door. Open the door slowly, quietly. Peer out. See nothing. Tiptoe out into the parking lot so we can see the rooftop. Crane necks. Stare into darkness. Flick on flashlight. See nothing. Worry about neighbors seeing us and thinking we're from McLouth, Kansas – country rubes new to the city and impressed with how tall the buildings seem to be here in the Big City of Lawrence, Kansas. So, we go back inside.

Repeat the exact same thing the next night. Then … that's it. Silence. Visits from Barred Owl are nevermore. He's had his say, and what he said was, "Get off your ass and come out here to see and feel the love that nature has to offer." Or something like that.

II

Message of the Owl: OK, so now Owl has called with his Song-of-the-Sirens … and I will obey his call to track him to his source, to try to unravel the fabric of his true spirit, to perhaps fall in love with the spirit of Owl. He will not be an easy bird to track down, his spirit will prove to be multi-layered. This is a bird with many stories to tell; many myths, superstitions, and true tales to parse. But so be it.

I will night-walk – I always liked the nights out raccoon hunting or night fishing or taking a short walk away from the tent. Perhaps I will have a chance to speak with Owl; perhaps not. But I will be seeking more than feathered owl in his physical presence; I will be searching for those symbolisms he represents, trying to render unto me that which only the spirit can comprehend.

Taking the path to find the real truth about owls in general, you come almost immediately to a fork in the road that offers you two choices; either choice is a path well-traveled by those before you. Will you take the path that leads to wisdom, magical/mythological intrigue, and spiritual growth? Or, will you walk the one that portends doom, despair, agony, and death? Perhaps the shadows of the night will help you decide: Wisdom? Death?

III

Re-Learning How to Walk: Thanks to the siren call of Hoot Owl, I begin my walking … because, after all, Motion Is Lotion. But there are other critters, other parts of nature, that will also be calling me, that also have lessons to teach. I will, After Cancer Diagnosis (ACD), try my best to learn how to listen to them and heed their teachings. I will learn how to include them as an integral part of my spirit, my cancer-infested spirit.

My first walks are just walking in circles around the parking lot, trying my best to avoid the hint of a sashaying prissy gait. In a few weeks I will graduate from government-issue walker to a sleek loaner-walker with four wheels and a place to sit.

Leaving the government-issue walker behind did cause a few sad moments. I'd come to rather enjoy the annoying sound of metal on the hard floor of a shopping center – a vibrating scritch-scratch that echoed fingernails on a blackboard. It was a sound I thought appropriate as I trudged my way through any of the local MegaMarts, acting like I was shopping.

Shortly after my second walker, I graduated to walking sticks … which gave me the luxury of standing up and being able to crane my neck around to see more of the surrounding nature.

IV

Seeds of the New Me: As walking becomes ever easier; and as I continue to recover from surgery and regain at least a smidgen of my previous mental and physical abilities; and as I learn how to use my walking sticks to support my wobbling gait; and since the owls have given me the hooted motivation to get off my ass; and since I'm sick and tired of watching dogs poop, and watching TV, and watching planes overhead, I think I am almost there … ready to begin a new life.

V

Heeding the Call: It is interesting that it was one of the winged-ones who coaxed me off the couch and into daily nature-walking – and it was a night-owl to boot. Also interesting is that the coaxing was not from a direct connection, but rather from the spoken hoot.

Before we moved to the city, we'd listened to the variety of night sounds we heard on our small farmstead – from coyote yipping, yapping, and then howling at the moon; to the creeketing, cricketing, sturrrumpping, thrumping of all sorts of insect and frog sounds; to the incessantly wail-like chirp of whip-poor-will, whip-poor-will, whip-poor-will. (One of my ways to get to sleep in the camping tent was to count the number of whip-poor-will calls in a row before the little bastardly sound-machine paused to catch his breath.)

Owl sounds are uniquely and hauntingly nighttime, and they seem to have the ability to send at least two different messages, perhaps many more. The two most common owl sounds we heard on our farm in the country were from two different owl species: the Great Horned Owl and the Barred Owl.

The Great Horned is the larger of the two, and you'd think he'd have the louder booming voice. But the smaller (and some would say, feistier) Barred Owl has a much more brazen shout.

The Great Horned's voice seems apologetic, barely audible, whispering, "Whoo, whoo, whoooo." It's almost as if he is trying to entice prey to his nest site with a softly comforting tune. Barred Owl is a distinct opposite. His cry reaches out to any and all in the far reaches of his neighborhood, "Who cooks for you? Who cooks for you? Who cooks for you nowww?" he demands to know.

VI

Owl Prowl: Sue and I have led several *"Owl Prowls"*, usually for a group of grade-school aged campers. On an owl prowl you wait until it's good and dark, you round up the kids, tell them to be absolutely quiet and that no one (except the leaders) is allowed to have any source of light, and you hike into the woods. Some very practiced birders can almost perfectly mimic common owl sounds. I, however, have a battery-operated bird-sound maker – one with owl sounds on it.

Once we're into the woods, away from lights, we all sit down, and I turn on my owl calls. With a little luck we'll attract a resident owl who wants to protect his territory, and he comes in with a vengeance, talons up, expecting a fight. The kids are typically too excited to stay quiet or to refrain from flicking on their lights they've been keeping, hidden away, stuffed into pockets. Chaos reigns.

Amazingly, Owl almost always stays perched in the treetop – at least until he gets bored with the whole scene. He sits there and glares down at those little squirming urchins crowded below. And, with just a little light, it will be easy to see the glow of those huge eyes, one on either side of his head, pointed straight forward much as our human eyes are.

An owl's eyes are perfect for nighttime hunting; their placement gives him binocular vision for depth perception, and the nighttime eye-glow comes from a reflective surface on the retina which allows for a better look-see in the dark.

In addition to these visual adaptations for night hunting, an owl's ears are placed asymmetrically which allows it to determine exactly where those subtle nighttime scratching sounds are coming from – those subtle, rodent-made scritchings that the owl hopes will lead him to tonight's meal. (And by the way, an owl's ears are located at the side of his head. Those ear-like thingies atop the Horned Owl's head are feather tufts, function unknown.)

An owl's face is also shaped like a satellite dish which allows it to concentrate sounds into a more acute audible reception.

In other words, owls come hard-wired to pick up tiny night sounds and to relay those sounds so that the owl's brain is given precise azimuth (both direction and height) information of its prey … much like the info provided by the Omni stations used by pilots.

If we're lucky on our owl prowl, Owl will sound off and give us some of his vocal repertoire – usually an angry series of hoots and hollers. Most often, though, he'll just sit there looking down quizzically, as if to say, "Who the hell do you think you are, down there, making a bunch of noise, keeping me from my hunting?"

If it's a Barred Owl that comes in to see us, the kids often think he looks a lot like Hedwig, Harry Potter's 11th birthday gift from Rubeus Hagrid. Although they do look similar, Hedwig is a Snowy Owl, not a Barred Owl. Snowy Owls are almost all white, while our Barred Owls distinct brown bars on a white background give him away.

Snowy Owls are only occasional wintertime visitors to our parts of the country, coming down from northern climes when hunting is poor up there. Finally, Hedwig's job is to deliver mail; our Barred Owl's jobs include catching little nighttime rodents … and maybe raiding an occasional chicken house.

VII

Last Words: So, owls are special emissaries of the nighttime, but real contact with *any* being of Nature has the potential for creating lasting impressions, far reaching impacts. It is with this in mind that I feel better prepared for the next phase of my life – chemotherapy.

Chapter 8 Interlude: Owl In the Henhouse

One morning, years ago, while doing chores on our farm outside of St. George, I opened the door to the chicken coop and there he was; a huge Great Horned Owl, sitting on the floor, looking confused. Evidently, he'd flown through a small window to the coop and then couldn't figure how to get out. Without an exit strategy, he'd abandoned his original plan to grab a chicken, and so he sat there, glaring at me.

I take my sweatshirt off with the idea of trapping him under it, and I move slowly toward him, circling to get around behind. This plan-of-attack doesn't work. He swivels his head to follow me, never taking his eyes off my approach. He fluffs his feathers, hoists his wings up to make him look like a ferocious linebacker, and he is ready to do battle with me. He hisses once, twice, then several times he clacks his bill, menacingly.

One of the folklores of owls is that you can keep circling them until they eventually wring their own neck ... and then you've got them. The reality is that owls have only one swivel point of neck-to-head contact – compared to our human heads that have two points of contact – which allows owls (and other birds) to swivel around to their actual physical limit which is usually about 270 degrees.

To help with their neck swivel, owls (and other birds) have muscular and arterial structures in their necks that don't tear apart with the stretching that comes from the head-turning. And finally, owls have 14 cervical (neck) vertebrae – birds, in general, have from 13 to 25 cervical vertebrae whereas all mammals have seven. (Think of that! From prairie vole to human to giraffe, all of us mammals are stuck with seven neck vertebrae.) These extra neck bones give birds the increased flexibility needed to reach around and then downward to preen the feathers on their body, back, and butt.

My owl's stare-down with me ends quickly when I get too close. He leaps into the air, takes off with a swoosh of wing-feathers, and … flies right into a corner where I easily toss the sweatshirt over his head. I pin his wings down underneath my sweat-shirt, make sure beak and talons are pointed out and away from me, carry him out of the hen house, march to the edge of our woods, throw him into the air, and he is up, up, and away.

Wait! What? Is that bird flipping me the feather? That middle primary on his right wing sure looks to me as if it's pointed straight up. "Well, screw you too", I holler as he disappears out of sight.

Note to self: Remember to shut the danged window to the henhouse from now on.

Hear Me Out

I

The Meet-Up: It's been about a month since my tumor-ectomy. Thanks to the hoot of an owl and the prodding of Sue (now known as Nurse Ratchet), I am out and about, walking – still wobbling, but almost upright – with the help of my walking sticks.

Sue is driving me to Kansas City, an hour away, for my first appointment with my oncologist. We were advised to wait for a month after the surgery before beginning chemo – apparently plenty long enough to make sure I don't croak from surgical "complications."

The most common complications from surgery (according to a handout from John Hopkins U.) include: shock, hemorrhage, wound infection, deep vein thrombosis and pulmonary embolism, other lung complications, urinary retention, and adverse reactions to anesthesia – including the most severe of all reactions: death.

An *oncologist* is a medical professional who practices a branch of medicine that deals with the prevention, diagnosis, and treatment of cancer. Oncology, from New Latin onco- ("tumor"), from Ancient Greek word ὄγκος (óngkos), meaning ("burden, volume, lump, mass, bulk"), and –logy, ("study of"). Oncology can be generally divided into 1. Medical oncology, 2. Radiation oncology, and 3. Surgical oncology.

II

KU Cancer Center: Cancer is such a colossal problem in our society that one of its local treatment centers, the *University of Kansas Cancer Center*, has, in just the last few years, taken over what was once a Sprint Center and has repurposed that bastion of capitalism into an entire "cash-cow hospital" with multiple floors (requiring chemo-fogged patients to remember where they are and where they are going … so they can push the correct elevator button), several separate areas of treatment (radiation, chemotherapy, and surgical), free parking (valet if you want it), and an old-style, walk-through cafeteria with attached patio (outdoor seating available).

Later on, while wandering aimlessly about, Sue and I will stumble onto the cafeteria. *The cafeteria* in the cancer hospital offers a couple of three-course, hi-carb, hi-fat dinners. Or you can munch on any of the many salty snack offerings; gulp one of several choices of soda pop or other sugary drinks.

Regardless of your choices, you will eat with plastic utensils, use plastic cups and plates to eat and sip off of, and carry your food to the table on plasticized trays – which will then be used to take the leftovers (including the now-used plastics) to the garbage cans. Garbage that will then be hauled to the already overfull city dump.

Apparently hidden from view in this cafeteria are any nutritionally healthy organic foods. Nor are there any foods or herbal seasonings that enhance the health of the intestinal microbiome or that have been shown to be effective against cancers or their common comorbidities. And there is a smoking area just outside on the patio.

III

Back to Day One at the KU Cancer Center: We pass through the portal of entry to the hospital, and a uniformed cop directs us to our first staging area. I suppose he's there to keep the cancer-ridden from stealing chemotherapy poisons … which must be hot items on the street nowadays.

Our first staging area is a large room, devoid of happy decor or positive energy. The reception-room's plastic chairs and couches are already fully occupied by a small herd of people, most of whom are either sitting abjectly in their seats with arms folded over their chest and rocking slowly. Or they sit silently slumped forward – their blank and tired stares focused on the carpet in front of them, a well-worn carpet, pock-marked with the coffee spillings and excretal stains from the still-living.

The building is only a few years old, and already it looks and feels decrepit, as if it needs major surgery.

When one of the three admittance receptionists is free, we go to her desk, answer the same list of questions that have been posed more than a gazillion times already, get two plastic wristbands – one with my name and birth date and a QR Code Reader that will let me pass through the checkout desk … as one more tally to the day's till.

The other wristband announces me as a *FALL RISK!* I like the *FALL RISK* bracelet as a prestige symbol, and so I make sure to keep mine on for as long as I can after each treatment.

This first staging area reminds me of the pens where cattle are grouped before they are driven through the treatment chute where they are castrated, ear tagged, vaccinated, given a dose of Ivermectin® wormer and any other medications deemed necessary to help them stay alive long enough to make it to the slaughterhouse.

I feel the urge to bawl like a calf that has lost his mamma, decide better, sit down, wait to be called to the vampire den where they will try to take my blood.

IV

The Vampire Den: In the "vampire den" I will be entertained by ladies who will fearlessly try to collect my blood. I am what is known by *phlebotomists* as a "tough stick." (Phlebotomists are people trained to draw blood; for vampires, drawing blood comes naturally.) My veins tend to collapse and roll whenever poked at. I'm usually a sweaty mess with arms full of painful punctures by the time I hear the vein-poker's sigh of relief and can (finally!) observe that thin line of red going from vein into the collection tubes.

Today, after several "dry wells", my phlebotomist eventually (finally!) hits blood. The blood will be sent to the lab where a bank of humming machines will take readings on the cells, minerals, and biochemicals – proteins, sugars, enzymes, and more – the stuff that's currently swimming around in the fluids of my blood.

The data that the machines have captured from the depths of my innards will be spit out as occult numbers which will magically appear as print-outs on 8″ x 12″ flat pieces of paper. These numbers, after being amalgamated and parsed by a team of people with lots of letters after their names, will then be used to diagnose, prognose, and devise a protocol for my treatments to follow.

Pretty amazing that they can do all this … without even once running their hands over me, examining my body – feeling for the flow of my energetics (or chi) and testing for areas of pain; without physically moving my joints to test for flexibility or mobility; without ever listening to the movements of any of my vital inner parts. Pretty amazing indeed.

I've had a shit load of the types of tests that are run by machines on various parts of my body. Someday I plan to paper my office walls with the printouts.

V

Hear Me Out: After the blood-letting, Sue and I are led to a different staging area, a gathering of more steers headed to slaughter. After reading every magazine available (all of which date back to the Inquisition), the nurse calls my name, checks my bracelets, asks me the same questions once again, then leads us to the exam room where we meet, for the first time, the good doctor, Doctor ABC, MD PhD (not his real name).

Dr. ABC, MD PhD is a pleasant young man, dressed in a loose-fitting suit with tie, tiny of stature, brown of skin, quiet of nature. He smiles and offers a polite handshake and looks at my chart. "Well, James," he says with a serious tone, "your PSA (Prostate Specific Antigen) has gone down quite a bit since the surgery. It was 5,065.43 before the surgery, and now it's back down to close to normal. And the MRI looks … and he drones on and on and on, explaining what the MRI showed about the condition of my innards.

But I am curious (and bored). I interrupt him and ask, "So how does my 5,065 compare to others you've seen?"

"Well, it's the highest I've ever seen, almost double the next highest," he answers matter-of-factly.[4]

---

4 PSA normal reference range varies with age. The normal reference range in a 75

Aha! Once again: I'm Number One! I'm Number One!! I think an Irish jig is in order, try to stand up, feel Nurse Ratchet's fingernails digging into my already-puncture-riddled arm, decide to stay seated.

Being a winner once again encourages me to give the standard talk that I give to all medical personnel: "Doc," I say, "we need to be perfectly clear on one thing; you are *not* here to keep me alive. You're here to help me maintain a decent quality of life ... for however much longer I have left."

In a lifetime of visiting various and sundry doctors, I've had only one doc who responded positively to this talk – and he was an old guy, a bit older than I was at the time, about to retire. He replied, "Well, I'll be damned. You're my kind of patient. I've always thought that's exactly what I want; quality of life, not just life everlasting."

I can hope. "So doc," I continue, "we both know that chemotherapies have a ton of adverse side effects, and, after all is said and done, they really don't give you much more time alive anyway."

To which he replies, "Hear me out, James, hear me out." (This is a refrain we will hear many times, repeated over and over again). After singing his refrain, he starts on a litany of reasons to sell me on the "fact" that the chemotherapy regime he recommends to patients is this generation's silver bullet – the wonder drug that is the best thing to happen to cancer patients since the discoveries of ether and formaldehyde.

According to Dr. ABC, MD PhD, side effects are only a small matter of concern: they are usually mild, they don't happen to all patients, and if you do have them, they don't last long. All this sounds vaguely familiar. Then I put it together. It's the exact same type of talk that, as a practicing veterinarian, I heard over and over again from the sales reps who called on me. Dr. ABC, MD PhD had memorized the sales rep's talk and was repeating it back to me ... as if I couldn't read the drug inserts with their long lists of adverse side effects for myself.

---

to 79 year old man (my age at the time of the surgery) varies – depending on who is doing the referencing – from 0.0 to 6.5 ng/mL or from 4.5 to 5.5 ng/mL or from 0 to 7.95 ng/mL, and normal values may range from 0 to 11.98 ng/mL in 80-84 year olds and up to 33.17 ng/mL in men 85 and older. And isn't it simply delightful that even the term "normal" can have such a variety of so many widely-differing definitions.

Dr. ABC, MD PhD has cast his line into my waters, expecting me to see only the wiggling minnow at the end of the line.

VI

Closing the Sale: Dr. ABC, MD PhD puts on his serious face – in order to, I suppose, sell me on his current concept of silver bullet. "James," he speaks in a barely audible whisper, "the normal lifespan projection for your level of cancer is about six months to a year. With treatment," he claims, "you may live for 4 to 5 more years. And during this time, you'll be able to function normally."

He finishes with a flourish, "I'll give you copies of the studies that show the data to support all this. And, if the treatments do make you sick, we can always stop them. Read the studies, think about it, and we can set up an appointment for you to begin in a few weeks." All this said with a smile and then a handshake.

Sue and I leave; drive home in silence.

VII

The First Remorse: At home, I scan the articles he has given me – the words melting into Rorschach blots on the page. Blots of ink that I find impossible to interpret.

It is only later, much later, that I re-read those same articles. And, with a more critical and in-depth reading (and with more time to think, really think, without the hum of hospital in the background), I discover the way the drug companies skewed the data to embellish their drug's results. And it's only later yet that, after going through several months of treatment, I know the real cost of the side effects one endures during treatment.

But by then, I have already swallowed the lure – hook, line, and sinker. And like the google-eyed walleye, I am flopping around on the shore … a fish out of water.

Chapter 9 Interlude: Why They Lie

I

Why They Lie: In a very interesting study,[5] we learn that most oncologists lie. In the study of patients with advanced cancer, 71% of the patients wanted to know the truth about their prognosis; only 17.6% of those want-to-know patients were told the truth by their oncologist. Most were given false hopes and far too optimistic expectations for the likely outcomes of treatment.

But why the lie? Oncologists all seem like such nice people, dedicated to saving lives. And they all have spent many years of their life, learning how to use today's best choice of silver bullet for thwarting the growing menace that cancer poses on our species.

So, what gives here? Well, as with most things in our current institutionalized world of reality, there are a slew of reasons for why oncologists lie, and most of them seem fairly reasonable… at first glance.

II

Hope: Hope is often given as the answer to "why I lie to my cancer patients" – as in: I lie to my patients to give them more hope, because: a) with a hopeful prognosis they will have a more positive attitude, and positive attitudes tend to contribute to more positive outcomes; b) with hope in their hearts, my patients will be more apt to have the heart and the guts to continue with the therapies I recommend, therapies that will be difficult to tolerate at best; c) hope springs eternal – which means that my hopeful patients will tend to continue with therapies even after it is apparent the hoped-for outcome is highly unlikely.

But, when patients are lied to about their prognosis (or just not told), they can hold unreasonable expectations and elect to participate in futile treatment plans that ultimately lower their

---

5 Enzinger Ac, et al., Outcomes of Prognostic Disclosure: Associations With Prognostic Understanding, Distress, and Relationship With Physician Among Patients With Advanced Cancer. Clin Oncol, 2015. 33(32); p. 3809-16. [PMC free article] [PubMed] [Google Scholar]

quality of life (QoL). Plus, patients who understand their prognosis are more likely to pursue treatments that better match their expectations, and they handle advance care planning such as living wills and do-not-resuscitate orders in a more timely manner.

Furthermore, when a patient is lied to about the likelihood and severity of adverse side effects of treatments, and when these side-effects eat into the patient's quality of life, that patient tends to lose all hope. Hopelessness is one of the biggest contributors to severe depression...and the resulting loss of quality of life.

And so, the two-edged sword of hope rears its ugly head.

III

Runaway Patients: Oncologists are aware that, if they tell their patients the real truth about their disease, its prognosis, and the hardships they might need to endure to go through treatment...they will likely leave – for another oncologist who is willing to offer more false hope.

An oncologist has spent 14 to 16 years[6] developing the skills to diagnose and treat cancer. After investing that much time and effort, every oncologist hopes to cure as many lives as he/she can. When those hopes and dreams are dashed because patients leave, it leads to doctor depression...and ultimately to a diminished quality of life for the oncologist.

IV

Capitalism: Far be it for me to even suggest that capitalism rears its ugly head in any doctor's thinking. Ever. However, capitalism is the overlying institution that controls almost every other institution in our current world.

And, even if it's not the oncologist who has capitalistic desires at heart, the Big Pharma Drug Lords who sell the cancer treatment drugs and the patient monitoring machines and the surgery instruments and the hospital beds and the nursing care that goes along with the beds and on and on...all these have a

---

6 Four years to get a bachelor's degree, followed by four years in medical school. Then medical oncology requires four to six years in an internal medicine residency. Many oncologists also spend a few more years in a fellowship.

heavy capitalistic hand in all exchanges between oncologist and patient. Patient Beware!!

V

Death and Dying: Capitalism may be the cloud that fogs all other institutions in our country, but our country's people and our attitudes also contribute to the fog. Particularly our attitudes about death – our deathly fear of death. As in: "Death? I don't even want to talk about it." And "Death and dying? Not for me? I plan to never die." And "Don't you ever bring up that topic to me again. You know it's bad luck to talk about death or dying."

And so, put yourself into the predicament of the oncologist. Many of their patients will not even want to talk about death or dying. Remember that about 30% of all cancer patients in one study didn't even want to hear what their prognosis was after they learned they had cancer.

Our willingness to acknowledge the inevitability of death or even to talk about it depends on our cultural background, our spiritual beliefs, our family's normal way of handling death-in-the-family, and perhaps even our level of education. How is the oncologist expected to parse all that out...so she/he can come up with an acceptable talk with the patient (and possibly the family member or other caregiver) about the terminal cancer the patient has. Not an easy task – made even more difficult by the seriousness of the situation.

Hear JR Kidd Out

I

Hear Me, Randy Kidd, Out: OK, after hearing "Hear me out, James, hear me out" dozens of times, I figure it's high time someone should listen to me. To moi. And by the way, I've never been "James", it's always been Randy.

And as another BTW, I do not typically use my doctor title … except I did enjoy demanding it from drug salesmen when I was in practice. (And, I do make Sue refer to me as "Doctor Doctor," but that's another topic for another time.)

The gist of this is that I want to be heard. I want to shout to the skies: "Hear *Me* Out," I want to have a say in those decisions that will affect whatever hours I have left, and I want my wants and life-preferences to enter into whatever decisions are made.

I understand it's difficult, if not impossible, to badger the impenetrable protocols that now oversee western oncology medicine – medical methods that have been generated by the monetary needs of today's cancer-care institutions. But I'm sick and tired of being given the sales talk about how great today's cancer treatments will be for me.

However, when you're dying of cancer, it's probably not the time to worry about trying to change any of the institutions our world has created.

And so, very early on (some of it written while I was still in the post-op recovery bed), I wrote down some of the principles I wanted to try to live by. Initially, I called them Randy's Manifesto – For Living With Cancer, but I later changed that to Yoda's admonition: **"Do Or Do Not. There Is No Try."**

II

Do Or Do Not. There Is No Try

- **Do Not A Burden Be.** Friends and family around me need to get on with their own lives … without having to worry about me. I need to quit whining, moaning, and groaning. Buck up. Man up. Step up! Deal with the realities as they come up. We're all dying; it's just that some of us are dying faster than others.

- **Motion Is Lotion:** *Keep Moving; Motion is Lotion, Rest is Rust; Movement is Medicine; Use It or Lose It; Move Every Joint, Every Day.* A daily walk, maybe some tai chi, chi gong, and/or yoga, and my prescribed physical therapy movements are must-dos. There are simply too many scientifically-proven health benefits to keeping the body in motion; there's no good reason to let body rust (and eventually the rust-of-cancer) take over.

- **Nature Heals.** I will *Move in Nature,* where the true healing energies exist. Walks, whenever possible, will be taken outside where I can see and feel what Nature has to offer. I need the winds of Kansas for their ability to sweep away the cobwebs of mind. And along the way I will talk to my four-legged, scaly, and winged natural healers. Happily, as I write this, some of them seem to be talking back.

- **Stay Creative:** Be as creative as possible – *Today and Everyday.* My form of creativity, my art form, is writing. (The six keys for being a successful writer: read, read, read; write, write, write.) I will continue writing until I am no more. Writing about Nature – Her inhabitants, and Her natural cycles – is my passion. I see cancer as one of nature's natural forces, and so I will be writing about it as such.

- **Love and Appreciate My Family.** To love and appreciate is not enough; I will do all I can to *show* them how much I truly love and appreciate them. I'm being given some time; I accept the challenge to determine how to best demonstrate my love and appreciation. This I will do despite living in a culture where it is often difficult to outwardly show love and appreciation.

- *It Is What It Is.* No woulda, coulda, shoulda for me! No sense replaying any of the possibilities that could have prevented the cancer or its progression, had I made life's decisions differently "back then." Today is; it is; and I am living in today time.

- **Defy Normals.** Two maxims I've tried to live by: John Lewis' "Get in good trouble" and another one I got from somewhere: "When you're known as crazy, it gives you a lot of leeway for behavior." No reason to shuck these now.

- **Seek Thin Places.** On my walks: stop, look and learn, listen and feel, respect. Search for those thin places in nature where earth seems to merge with the skies – places where spirits call and where the human mind can be wholly activated. Think thick thoughts while stopping, seeking.

- **Wonder-full Curiosity.** What are the life lessons cancer can teach me? Open up my mind and learn all I can – about cancer, about living well, about living as a part of nature, about how to die well, and more.

- **Time Is Ticking.** But, I have been given some small fragment of time: Time to get my affairs in order, time to tell the people I love how much I really love them and how proud I am of them, time to live out the tenets of my Do Or Do Nots. Thank you, Creator, for every instant of the time you have given me.

- **Appreciate**, really appreciate all that has been and continues to be given me. I am, and have been, truly blessed, and perhaps, just maybe, this cancer is another blessing in disguise.

- **Tao and Yin-Yang:** I use the Tao, and Yin-Yang – the basic principles of nature, nuance, and complementary/contradictory forces in our universe – as my fundamental and overriding guides.

- **Decisions, Decisions.** Many of them may not be easy … but they will have to be made. By me. Maybe after listening to others' concerns and other scientific evidence … but the buck stops with me. I will be the ultimate decision maker.

- *Illegitimi Non Carborundum (Don't let the bastards get you down)* Bastards come in many forms: rogue cells that are intent on growing amok despite the damage they cause to other cells; well-meaning cancer "experts" who want to infuse me with all sorts of poisons so I'll live longer (but not necessarily better); pain receptors that seem to be intent on firing off randomly and with intensities I've not experienced before; and more. I will not let any of these bastards get me down. Ever.

- **Wabi Sabi:** I will consistently adhere to the principles of Wabi Sabi … no matter how much hectoring I get from Sue: "Will you please clean up your damned office? Today?"
- **Teamwork Is How It Works.** It will take a team effort to, as John Wayne said: "Whup the Big C." I will keep my family, my extended family, and any friends who have become team members up to date on: 1) what science tells us about the current status of my cancer; 2) what my next options are; and 3) how I plan to deal with those options. I will also coach an integrated team of cancer therapists – a team that may include general practitioners, oncologists, surgeons, radiologists, physical therapists, and holistic practitioners of alternative medicines – so that we are all on the same page when it comes to how we will deal with my trickster-of-a-disease we call cancer.
- **I Rule.** *I am the captain of this ship* that I call my body, and I chart its courses, weather its storms, steer it according to my inclinations, and decide when it's time for the captain to abandon ship.
- **Have Fun.** The Irish in me will make this an easy tenet to live up to.
- **Overlying It All:** Both the keystone and the foundation of my basic life's mission: *"Reuniting the Human Spirit with the Soul of Nature."*
- **Finally,** *Die with Dignity, Peace, and Grace.* Death: just another stop on the natural cycles of life.

End of Do List

And so, I have some mottos, slogans, or old saws to cut a new pathway now that I have cancer; some ideas for how to live my life – my Do List. But as I review my List, I realize it's too much for me, at my age, to remember. And so I condense it into four major legs – legs I should be able to keep in mind for doing on a daily basis: *1) walk every day that I can stand up; 2) walk in Nature; 3) create something fantastic with my writing; and 4) honor my family.*

I remember that my first BIG Do was to not be a burden, a Do I also realized was nigh-on impossible. But maybe, just maybe – if I could put a collar on me, and if I handed the leash to a competent caretaker – someone like my Sue – then maybe my "me-walker" could control me enough that I wouldn't be a total burden. Maybe.

Finally, the tail that wags *this* dog is my life's motto: *"Re-uniting the Human Spirit with the Soul of Nature."*

III

The Fine Print: How's all this working for me now, almost five years into treatment? So far, I'm doing OK, following the principles of my Do List. Not great, and far from perfect, but most of the time I listen to the advice my list gives me. I find a certain amount of solace from the fact that really good baseball hitters get a hit less than a third of their times at-bat.

I do realize that – without defining the written terms **and** the actions it will take to carry them out, any manifesto (or list of values or principles or whatever you want to call those written words) – can very easily degenerate into blackboard bullshit. (Blackboard bullshit is that list of trite little sayings that coaches tack onto locker room walls and chalk on to blackboards – the kind of BS they use to excite ballplayers into 30 seconds of unbridled pre-game frenzy … and the kind of BS that, without firmly defined action steps, means nothing to anyone.)

IV

Last Words: Note to me: Any list of core principles needs to be re-evaluated periodically … so that I can tell if my actions are following my values. And so I can assess whether or not my actions are getting the results I want. And so I can compare my today's values against those that were important to me last year or last month.

In other words, the two keys to an effective list of core principles are 1) What does this principle actually *mean to me,* and 2) How will following this principle *impact* the way *I* live *my* life.

Chapter 10 Interlude: Manifesto Or??

I began writing my *Do Or Do Not* List thinking it should be called a manifesto. I liked the way Martin Luther's Manifesto created sweeping changes to stoic and staid (and highly profitable) religious institutions back in his day. And the way he pursued a fine figure of a woman, she a nun nonetheless. And how – in a fit of religious fervor – good old Marty was able to swift her away from the nunnery in a pickle barrel. And Marty's thirst for a good brew – he being so thirsty he taught his x-nun/now-wife how to run a brewery. And finally, the way good old Marty wrote his manifesto in a fury and supposedly nailed it to the door of a church.

Which was what I wanted to do initially: write a manifesto while still trying to deal with my cancer diagnosis … and then nail it to my office door so I could see it whenever I entered. But then Sue said I couldn't nail <u>anything</u> to *any* of *her* doors. Thus endeth that idea.

And besides, manifestos are usually written in a state of bowel-boiling agitation, the author wanting to change some aspect of society in general. Furthermore, manifestos are often penned as a want-list aimed at some group of others – with directions to *them* for what *they should* be doing to improve themselves.

My Do List might actually be an anti-manifesto in that it applies to me and me alone. It is only my plea to Self to improve myself … because I've been granted the time and (so far) the energy to do just that.

Part and parcel of my To Do List is that it was written as my personal vehicle to help me return my inner-most thoughts back to love – back to the love of nature, to the love of family, and ultimately to the love of Self. I have no skin in the game of trying to change others to my personal way of thinking.

Last Words: I do think that everyone, no matter their age or current health status, could benefit from writing down their own self-directed To Do List of core principles … before they are no longer able to.

From Henry David Thoreau: *"Pursue some path, however narrow and crooked, in which you can walk with love and reverence."*

Spider Webs

I

Spiders have taken the Art of Living to a new level, a level that some of us might need to use a squinty-eyed look-see to appreciate. After walking through a game trail draped with dozens of spider webs and having to wipe those infernal sticky filaments off brow and out of nostrils and mouth, most of us are not inclined to think kindly thoughts about the maker's art form.

(One cure for the spider-web-on-game-trail malady is to convince your spouse – or any newbie walker – that it is a great privilege to lead the hike … then let them clear the way for you.)

Spiders are, in fact, another of those creatures capable of conjuring wide extremes of human emotion. Some (more pragmatic) folks admire spiders for their "art-eye" and their "carpentry" skills and for their patient prowess as hunters-in-lurk that helps keep unwanted bug populations down. Other folks are scared to death of them – arachnophobia (severe fear of spiders) effects from 3 to 15% of the population and is often listed in the top ten of all the fears we humans have.

Still others have made the spider into a variety of symbolic images – from spiritual to spooky, from the wily trickster to the patient and persistent hunter, from the exemplar of wisdom to the harbinger of the curse, and from being associated with death to being a part of the culture's origin story. Finally, in today's world, spider and his web have inhabited many of today's cultural symbols, from the World Wide Web to the heroic Spider-Man.

From cultural symbolism, to pragmatic appreciation, to absolute fear and loathing, the spider has certainly attracted our attention.

II

Iktome: Iktome is a shapeshifter (able to appear as a human figure) and a spider-trickster in Lakota mythology. Like most tricksters, Iktome offers us continuing lessons of how to use wisdom for making our decisions … while at the same time trying to trick us into looking so foolish others will laugh at us for our folly.

Iktome – often working in union with Coyote, another shape-shifting trickster – is involved in stories that try to teach us to behave honorably and help us avoid trouble by thinking critically about situations. Iktome is always teaching us about the consequences of our actions, and she is also famous for using strings to control humans like puppets.

III

Spider Webs: Not all spiders weave webs. Some, like the wolf spider for example, quietly stalk their prey, chase it down if necessary, and then pounce on it much like, well, much like the wolf does.

But, of the web weavers there are four major forms of webs they weave: 1) funnel-shaped webs (these are mostly found low to the ground), 2) tangled or cobwebs (commonly found in dark, unused spaces around the home), 3) sheet web (dense flat or bowl-shaped layers of silk), 4) orb weavers (perhaps the most familiar, a web made into spokes of a wheel with a spiral design between spokes).

When we speak of a web of artistic merit, we are generally referring to the orb weaver's web, an intricate design of structural beauty that, after a dewy night, glistens and almost glows in the morning's light.

> *Imagine a multidimensional spider's web*
> *in the early morning covered with dew drops*
> *And every dew drop contains the reflection*
> *of all other dew drops --*
> *And so on ad infinitum*
> *That is the Buddhist conception of the universe in an image*
> *— Alan Watts, Following the Middle Way*

Look a little closer and you'll see that the web is also a structure of functional integrity: 1) it is made from filamentous strands of sticky, bug-entangling silk, spun by the spider and shot like a bullet through its rear-aimed spinnerets; 2) the spokes and interweaving connectors are placed so that the weaver-spider can navigate them without getting stuck herself; and 3) the silken strands have more tensile strength than steel.

Spiders have been spinning silk since they emerged from the oceans some 400 million years ago. Over the years spiders have been developing specific types of silk with multifunctional uses that include: 1) wrappings to keep captured prey for another day; 2) a screen to hide behind; 3) as a long-stranded "parachute" that is spun and cast to the winds … so they can latch on and travel to faraway places; and 4) as a mate or prey attractor (some silks include the pheromonal scent that a male spider finds irresistible; other silks use pheromones to attract prey).

IV

Spider Bites: Nearly all spiders have venom glands, and a bite from almost any spider can cause some pain and even allergic reactions in susceptible people. However, only a few species can be a serious threat to humans – in our area of the world (Kansas) there are three of these: the Black Widow, the Brown Recluse and the Brown Widow. Any of these can cause from mild to significant tissue damage at the site of the bite, and some bites may cause major allergic reactions that could be life-threatening.[7]

---

7   The bad news is that some spiders do bite people, and these bites can be dangerous. The good news is that spider bites are actually quite rare events. A recent summary of reported spider bites in the United States between 1989 and 1993 included fewer than 5,000 incidents per year. Only a few of the bites of widow spiders were medically serious, but over 80% of recluse bites were considered serious. Only about 10% of other spider bites had serious consequences.

These numbers seem small when compared to the over 800,000 dog bites that required stitches each year (source: Centers for Disease Control). During the study period, dog bites were responsible for 20 deaths per year, and auto-deer collisions were associated with 130 annual deaths. There were no reports of spider-bite related fatalities during that four-year period.

Furthermore, the reality is that many injuries that are reported as spider bites are actually caused by other small animals (fleas, lice, mosquitoes, biting flies, ant bites and stings, etc.). One national study of 600 cases of suspected spider bites established that approximately 80% were not actually caused by spiders. (*Spider Bites*, The Ohio

V

My Spider Bites: I've never, to my knowledge, been bitten by a spider. Thanks be to the Nature gods, or to me Irish good luck … or to the fact that we've had indoor plumbing wherever we've lived. (Lots of Black Widow bites have been delivered to human butts, tantalizingly protruding through the hole in an outhouse – a favorite hangout for that spider species.)

I have the vague feeling, however, that I am in the midst of experiencing something akin to one or more of the spidery trapping methods I've seen in nature.

My spidery web is the web of marketing threads woven by BigPharm, and it is, perforce:

1) A work of artistic merit

2) A highly structured campaign, designed to fill the coffers of the industrial Fat Cats. The campaign includes: artistically deceptive ads placed on multiple media outlets, doctor shills – many of whom have been paid enormous sums for their testimonials, and sweet-young-thing drug reps who call on unsuspecting doctors.

3) Like the spider web, BigPharma's web is constructed of materials that are plenty strong enough to wrap me in its clutches and hold me there … until it has devoured and digested me.

Come into my parlor, said the spider to the fly.
– poem by Mary Howitt (1799–1888), published in 1829

"Oh what a tangled web we weave
When at first we begin to deceive"
– 19th century Scottish author Sir Walter Scott,
From: Marmion: A Tale of Flodden Field

VI

Germ Theory of Disease: But, as I worry about my own susceptibility to being lured into the spider's parlor, I realize that Western Medicine lured patients into its parlor long before I was born. The Germ Theory of Disease has, in just the last 150 years

State University, Marion March 28, 3021.)

or so, become the primary way Western Medicine approaches disease in general.

Fathering the Germ Theory of Disease were two main characters: Robert Koch (1843 – 1910) and Louis Pasteur (1822-1895). Koch established that a particular germ could cause a specific disease. Koch developed a list of four criteria that were used to determine that a certain germ caused a particular disease. Integral to these criteria is Postulate #3: "The disease must be reproduced when a pure culture is inoculated into a healthy, susceptible host."

Pasteur further proved that bacteria caused infection and disease – and went on to develop the use of weakened germs to make vaccines. He also developed pasteurization.

Following in the footsteps of these two, Paul Ehrlich (1854-1915) developed "antibiotics" that attacked the germs. He also warned, early on, about the possibility for these antibiotics to be toxic to humans, and that, additionally, it was likely that the germs would eventually find a way around the antibiotics.

While the Germ Theory has led to many advances in medicine, it has also led to a medical system hogtied to the limits of one-dimensional thinking … an institutional system which can only see disease through the lens of "one germ, one treatment." The seed of the Germ Theory has thus been used to grow a vast plantation of monoculture thinking – resulting in the idea of the "silver bullet" as the cure-all for all our medical concerns.

Last Words: As I think about Iktome, I am reminded that it was only a few weeks ago when, like a walleyed fish, I was hooked and then yanked out of my previous watery comfort zone … where, for several decades I had been relying on holistic methods to treat whatever ailments lay before me.

That was the preamble to this story, a story that will now shift from decision making to acting upon the decisions. It's a story that flips from a watery environment into the breeze in the trees – where Iktome-the-spider has built his web.

But the morals to the story are the same: think critically to make wise decisions, actions have consequences, realize that Iktome can string you along like a puppet … making you look as foolish as a walleye out of water.

Chapter 11 Interlude: Silver Bullets

I

Silver Bullets: It takes a silver bullet to kill a werewolf. This, a not-so-well-known "fact" (more fiction than fact) from the mid-1700's story wherein the hunter, Jean Chastel, killed the man-eating Beast of Gevaudan with bullets made by melting down the medals of the Virgin Mary he wore on his hat and then forming them into bullets.

(Strange how Christianity and werewolves seem to be so frequently woven together in the stories of yore, often as a way to separate man from nature.)

Then, two centuries later, along comes the masked man, declaring: "Come on, Silver! Let's go, big fellow! Hi-yo, Silver! Away!" (Silver was the Lone Ranger's second horse, following his first, named "Dusty." Like any good veterinarian, I wonder whatever became of Dusty.)

Silver (the horse) was transportation for the man carrying the Silver Bullets, symbols of justice, law and order: the Lone Ranger, a paragon of virtue for his time.

You could say that werewolf-susceptible-to-silver-bullet and Silver Horse/silver bullet were the mythological lead-ins for scientist, Paul Ehrlich to conjure the initial concepts that led to today's idea of the silver bullets of medicine...or in Ehrlich's terminology the **"magic bullets"** of medicine. In Ehrlich's words: "those medicines constrained by charm to fly straight to their specific objective and to turn aside from anything else in their path."   Ehrlich was speaking of natural antibiotics – the highly targeted medical treatments that he was in the process of developing.[8]

---

8 Ehrlich's initial "magic bullet" (in German: zauberkugel) was an arsenical compound directed toward treating syphilis; it was also known as compound 606 (chemically arsphenamine), the drug he had used to treat a syphilis infected rabbit in the early 1900's. Compound 606 eventually became the trade-named "Salvarsan," and it replaced the treatment of the times for syphilis – 2 to 4 years of painful and toxin-laden mercury injections. But Salvarsan's arsenic ingredient also proved to be more toxic than desired...and so was replaced with the less toxic Neosalvarsan – the magic bullet used to treat syphilis until the arrival of penicillin toward the middle of the 20th century.

It should be noted that several scientists (including Ehrlich and Alexander Flemming, he of penicillin fame, and both of whom worked on the early-on development of magic bullets, warned us that they might not be so magical after all: 1) they almost always brought to the patient a list of adverse side effects – allergic reactions, anaphylaxis and more; and 2) they only lasted so long before the "germ" figured a way to get around their lethal effects.

For example, nowadays, according to CDC, more than 2.8 million antibiotic resistant infections occur in the U.S. each year and more than 35,000 people die as a result. Penicillin has become, over the years, the drug that causes the most allergic reactions – 8 to 12% of the population, according to at least one reference are allergic to penicillin.[9]

And to bring this closer to home: my cancer cells, after they have initially been killed off by chemotherapy, will eventually figure out a way to circumvent whatever therapy we throw at them – and end up, once again, feasting on my bone and organ cells...until I have no more living cells to feed them.

For the most part, we have totally ignored the early-on warnings of the scientists. And why does that not surprise me?

9 Allergy Asthma Proc. 2014 Nov-Dec. 35(6): 489-494; Prevalence and characteristics of reported penicillin allergy in an urban outpatient adult population. Stephanie Albin, M.D. and Shradha Agarwai, M.D.

My First Chemo

My First Chemo: It was with some degree of trepidation that we made our appointment to begin chemo, but here we are. I take a small amount of comfort from the realization that the silver bullet my onco-doc recommends is derived from a product of nature: Taxol, the active ingredient of Docetaxel®, is the chemo-drug they will be injecting into my veins – it is a derivative of extracts from the bark of the Pacific yew (or western yew), *Taxus brevifolia,* a medium-sized evergreen, native to the Pacific Northwest.

It is ***not*** so comforting to know that all parts of many plants in the *Taxus spp* are poisonous to almost all species, including the human species … capable of causing death when ingested, and also capable of creating severe allergic reactions in some people. Even exposure to the pollen can be highly allergenic to some people, and experts believe that on-going allergies to the taxol-containing drugs may be due to previous exposure to the pollen, writ large in the clouds of springtime tree pollen wherever yews grow.

Nor is it comforting to realize that what will be injected into my veins is not directly from the tree, but rather has been brewed up in the caldrons of one of the BigNamePharmas. This means that the drugs circulating through me will have the ***appearance on paper*** of one of the yew tree's chemicals deemed to be the silver bullet by the chemists … but they will not be from the tree nor exactly as Nature intended them to be.

Would it be any more comforting to know that evergreens often symbolize immortality and everlasting life – this from their own long life span and because they never lose their needles of green? Or should I be more concerned about the mythology that places the yew at the junction of death and rebirth? I do know for sure that the yew tree in Nature does not look anything at all like a bullet.

II

To the Treatment Room: Sue and I are back at the University of Kansas Cancer Center, going through the same rigamarole that gets me entered into the hospital's daily till. I am directed into the same vampire den where the phlebotomist draws blood and leaves an indwelling catheter in my vein – the entry portal where the chemotherapy nurses will eventually hook me up and let the gravity of the earth drip the chemo-poisons into my veins.

Before we are herded into the IV therapy area of the cancer center, we will meet briefly with my onco-doc, Doctor ABC, MD PhD, who reassures me: "James, this is the very best thing we could possibly do for your condition."

We are then ushered through another door, walked down a long hallway, and are pointed to a room with a recliner (for me) and a stiff-backed chair (for Sue), a TV, and we are asked if we want warm blankets and perhaps coffee and something to munch on. All very friendly.

Recliners: Overstuffed, oversized, chairs meant to let you sit back and relax. Watch TV. Sip coffee or an adult beverage. Perhaps get a massage by flipping a switch on the recliner. High-priced recliner models can be asked to warm you while they are massaging.

While I was with the volunteer fire department, we were called out to a residence where the caller thought his elderly mother had just died. Possible Code Black. It was an early morning call, so the only two responders available were Chief Jay and me.

It did turn out to be a Code Black: silver-haired lady, no pulse, already cooled to room temperature, still in nightgown and robe, looking comfortable in her recliner, a nearby table holding coffee cup and cinnamon roll, and the TV still blaring Fox News.

As we worked the run, checked with the live-in adult son, and called the required officials, Jay waved me over: "See that," he said gravely, "Damned recliners. I swear they are a prime cause of death. Almost every Code Black I've ever run has someone in a recliner. I won't allow one of those god damned things in my house."

Since that day with the Code Black lady in the recliner, neither will I … but here I am in the treatment room, sitting in a recliner. Actually, I find it very comfortable.

III

Chemo Poisons: My chemo-poison, Docetaxel, will eventually arrive. Docetaxel belongs to a class of chemotherapy drugs called plant alkaloids, and it is one of the antineoplastic cytotoxic medications. Most antineoplastic drugs (including Docetaxel) are classified by NIOSH (National Institute for Occupational Safety and Health) as hazardous drugs. *Hazardous drugs* are capable of causing serious effects including <u>cancer</u>, organ toxicity, fertility problems, genetic damage, and birth defects.

Our nurses wear disposable Hazmat gowns as protection from the Docetaxel poisons; Sue and I are not offered one. We are also not told that it is not known whether chemotherapy drugs can be passed to your partner through bodily fluids. Because of this, the recommendation is to use a condom for vaginal or anal sex or a dental dam for oral sex for at least 48 to 72 hours after treatment. Nice to know.

Along with my Docetaxel I get a dose of I.V. corticosteroids … so that I have a reduced chance to croak while reacting to the poisons.

IV

Adverse Side Effects: Reactions to chemo drugs (actually to almost all drugs) are, depending on who you ask, relatively uncommon (so says Big Pharma and the onco-folks), or relatively common (if you're one of those worry warts who consider small percentages of say 5% of patients treated—but maybe up to 30% —as relatively common). Reactions to drugs (listed on the package insert as **"adverse side effects"**) occur either in response to something in the drug itself or as a result of an activation of the body's immune system.

To be sure, most reactions are mild: soreness (at the injection site or generalized muscle aches and pains), fever, skin rash, headache, etc. But reactions may be severe and even life-threatening.

Anaphylaxis is a serious reaction, rapid in onset (usually in a matter of minutes or hours), that may cause death. Common causes include insect bites, foods, and **medications**. Other causes include latex and extreme exercise … and anaphylaxis may also occur without any obvious reason.

Anaphylaxis typically causes more than one of the following symptoms: an itchy rash, throat or tongue swelling, shortness of breath, vomiting, lightheadedness, and low blood pressure. Treatment includes injection of epinephrine (thus making the EpiPen® a famous carry-along for many) … with follow-up therapies as needed.

Anti-cancer drugs are one of the medications known for their ability to cause comparatively high numbers of anaphylactic reactions – depending on several factors including the drug and the dosage used, reactions may occur in fewer than 1% of patients or up to as high as 10% of those treated.

The taxanes in use today, as a general category of chemo-drugs (that includes my docetaxel and also paclitaxel, a chemo-drug for treating mammary cancers), produce adverse reactions in about 10% of patients, and some of these result in life-threatening anaphylaxis.

The product label for docetaxel includes a black box warning of **toxic deaths, hepatotoxicity, neutropenia, hypersensitivity reactions and fluid retention**, with rates of death ranging from 0.6% to 2.8% of patients, the highest risk in those with preexisting liver test abnormalities.

V

Corticosteroids: Medicinal corticosteroids, because they ease swelling and irritation, are often used to treat conditions such as asthma, hives or lupus … or to help prevent aberrant immune-system reactions that may occur when some drugs are given. Today's cancer patients are typically given corticosteroids, along with the chemo-drugs, in order to minimize immune-related reactions.

The good thing about corticosteroids given along with chemo drugs is that they give you a false sense of feel-good, almost a buzz-like high. The bad thing about this is that the feel-good high is a false one. It makes you think you're getting better … when you are only feeling good for as long as you are still taking them.

Worse yet, **corticosteroids** also have a litany list of **adverse side effects**, including: increased risk of infections, diabetes, osteoporosis, weakening of tendons, mood or behavioral changes, skin and muscle atrophy, weight gain, facial swelling, depression, cramps, nausea and vomiting and other stomach irritation, bone fractures … ad infinitum.

Wait? What?? Isn't my cancer known for causing osteoporosis and bone fractures? And don't I want to continue to walk for as long as I am able – to help prevent bone fractures? And won't tendon weakening and weight gain make it more difficult for me to walk? And doesn't having cancer itself often cause severe mental problems … without adding depression, mood or behavioral changes, weight gain, and nausea and vomiting and stomach irritations to the mix?

Will you walk into my parlor? said the oncologist to me. 'Tis the prettiest little parlor you ever did see.

VI

Post Chemo: After reclining in my pretty parlor for an hour's worth of IV infusion (chemo and corticosteroids), I am patting my back with glee: I have survived, great god, I have survived. No anaphylactic crisis leading to death, not even a mild allergic reaction.

Sue and I decide to go to Lunner – a meal, popular with members of our family, that occurs frequently for us, in that gap between lunch and dinner. It's our way of celebration, the first treatment done and gone. Behind us.

But hell's fire, I don't need to add to the celebration my body is already feeling: the cortisone has kicked in. I'm feelin' – Hot Dam!! – I'm feelin' just fine and dandy, thank you very much. Floatin' on cloud nine, bein' hoisted (perhaps by angels) to the top of the towering cumulonimbus.

VII

Last Words: The cortisone high will last until the effect of the three-days-of-pills I've been given wears off ... about three days and a few hours from now. I am reminded of the tales chemo survivors have told me: "Hell, doc, the chemo was the easiest part of the treatment. I never felt better than when I was getting those IV drips. It was the days afterward that weren't worth a dam. Don't know how I survived those days."

It will only be during those "after days" when I will hear the siren call of "Will you walk into my parlor? It's the prettiest parlor you ever did spy," coming from a spidery voice somewhere in the bushes. Iktome in his wisdom mode? Or Iktome as puppeteer?

As I move toward the siren call, I will be caught in the invisibility of sticky web filaments. The spider watches calmly as I writhe and twist, knowing full well I am only getting myself further stuck. Stuck in a treatment regime I will not be able to free myself from ... perhaps until I die.

Oftentimes, after my walks in the woods, two thoughts cross my mind in perpendicular fashion: 1) how could I have possibly missed seeing the spider web? and, 2) In this game of life there are do-overs ... but not very damned many of them.

Chapter 12 Interlude: Consciousness and Soul Retrieval

I

Losing Consciousness: So now I've been cold-cocked *and* anesthetized, and I've endured my first chemo treatment, *and* I've survived all these unscathed. Or so I am thinking. What is yet to come is the swallowing of the soul that often accompanies chemo therapies. *AND...*

II

Soul Loss and Soul Retrieval: There is another side to this having your consciousness taken away from you, no matter the instigator. In the shamanic tradition soul loss is an important component of disease, and one way a person's soul can leave his body is during the time he is unconscious.

In some traditions, a person has several souls, each of which can be lost at various instances of body trauma, especially when the trauma induces coma. When your last soul is lost, that's the end of the road for you. Or so it is said.

Soul retrieval is thus an integral part of shamanic healing. Soul retrieval often takes the form of a journey to another world, another dimension.

III

The Shamanic Journey[10]: is taken after a body cleanse using the smoke of a sage or cedar or sweetgrass smudge and with the help of rhythmic drumming that resonates with the beating heart. In some traditions, this inner journey may be enhanced by "greasing" it with hallucinogenic drugs.

Oftentimes, a shamanic journey connects the patient with a power animal that can help with the healing process and perhaps show the patient how to reconnect with a lost soul. One shamanic technique helps the journeyer find his or her power animal that can then travel with the person for a lifetime, acting as protector along the way.

Most people have one power animal that is their personal link between their own inner powers and the powers of the supreme beings; some people are given many animals to travel with.

While journeying, power animals, acting as agents of healing, typically do not speak in full-sentence English. Rather, they of-

---

10 To make it perfectly clear: I do *not* consider myself a shaman. I've been fortunate enough to have worked with some people who I consider shamans, and I have learned from them. Over the years I have personally found using shamanic techniques as being very helpful.

fer some symbol, or they act out some story meant to symbolize what they are trying to tell you. You are then left to interpret the story or the symbol … always within your own frame of mind and current circumstances.

I'm a fan of the way shamanic healing and shamanic soul retrieval helps you, the patient, create your own reality. Perhaps it's this type of reality we should try to access whenever we've lost and then regained consciousness – no matter the cause.

IV

Last Words: For some folks the fear of death is the uppermost worry on their daily list of concerns. For others, death and dying is a constant haunting – a fierce predator, lying in wait somewhere around the next bend of life.

I am neither of these. For me death and dying are merely one more phase of life – hopefully a life well spent.

And I believe that, in order to spend one's life well, it's important to live it to the fullest. It's important to feed one's spirit and soul with all the positive energy and joy you can muster. I'm much more afraid of losing my spirit and soul than I am of arriving at death; for me death is simply the ending cycle of a life, lived alive.

PART THREE: GIFTS

Coming of Age Story

Coming of Age: I attended high school in the 60's in Lancaster, Ohio; a town about 30 miles southeast of Columbus. Lancaster offered only a few ways to craft your coming of age story: 1) Girls – I was a total klutz when around anyone wearing a skirt; 2) Cars – I couldn't tell a Porter from a Smitty, a mortal sin in an age of car love, bolstered with an ear for loud, popping car-sounds; or 3) Football – Lancaster is only a short 30 mile drive from the citadel of all things football: *The* Ohio State University.

For Ohioans football is not a way of life; it is life itself.

My dad and I had the usual father-son squabbles, but to my mind they mostly centered around his thinking that I was not being man enough, not tough enough for who he wanted me to be.

So, I set out to prove him wrong, of course, and I decided playing football might be my ticket to tough-guy status. I did not meet the "eye test" for the normal footballer of the day. I was a skinny, six- foot-one, 175 pound weakling. Almost anyone on the beach could kick sand in my face back then … which may have been the real reason I chose football as my storyline. But here's where I got lucky.

I had some natural speed (not white-lightning speed, but fast enough to win some high school hurdle races), and I had a fair amount of pain tolerance (thank you Irish genes). And, I really liked to hit people (thanks again Irish genes) … so football it was: my story of the struggle for how to come of age.

Apparently, there was enough of me to get a scholarship offer to play football at Iowa State University – true, it was not The Ohio State University, football's epitome (and the school where my dad had graduated). But ISU had a football team that played in what was then the Big 8 … again, not OSU's Big 10, but I figured it was good enough for me and my coming of age story.

On my recruiting visit to Ames, they walked me through the doors that connected the locker room with the playing field. Above the doors was a sign: "Through These Portals Pass the Hardest-Nosed Football Players In the World."

Sign me up!

That's how it all started. Back then we had a freshman team with two games on our schedule (we lost them both), and I was good enough to start at the end of my sophomore year. In those days you played both defense and offense, so in a typical game, I'd be out there on the field for 40 minutes or more … hitting guys, running pass routes, having fun.

I tell people I was a mediocre player on a mediocre team … because that's how it was.

II

"Awards": I got the game ball for the Virginia Military Institute (VMI) game – I think it was because that was the game where I got my three front teeth knocked out, and captain Dave felt sorry for me. I still have the blanket we were awarded as seniors – now moth-eaten and a much-faded cardinal and gold. Stitched onto the blanket are the four games when I was named lineman of the week. Today, I remember nothing about those games, including how I played in them.

Other "awards": two worn and torn shoulders – one that I can barely lift overhead (on a good warm day), and the other that is almost totally immobile. Bone spurs on almost every joint – chronic wear and tear. A total upper dental plate – three teeth knocked out cleanly, the rest gone as a result of poor dental work, bar brawls, etc.

More awards: Drug tolerance – at least that's what I call it. One game I was told I was the winner … for most pre-game novocaine® injections the team doctor had ever given to one guy. I was also taking one or two Darvon or Darvocet opioid painkillers every three hours during the season.[11] In addition, so I could sleep through the pain, at least two Seconal (sleeping pills), one

---

[11] It was only later that the Darvon drugs were declared to be "the worst prescription drug ever invented" – far too many suicides as a result of bad trips; plus they were not very good as pain killers anyway. In my case, whatever addiction I had to pain killers – liquid and capsular – I was fortunate enough to kick the capsular one, still working on the one that involves beer.

before bed, the other at about 3 am when the pain would wake me up.

Still more awards/benefits received: Bouts of heavy-duty depression throughout my lifetime – depression I attribute to all those many hits I took to the head. Four years of college paid for ... although in a moment of snit I figured out how much per hour we were making, figuring in all our time at practice, weight training, meetings, etc.: It came to about 25 cents per hour.

Nice job if you can get it. Ha!

The biggest benefit I got – and it was huge – was that Sue and I got married between my freshman and sophomore years. Plus, two of our three daughters were born while we were in Ames. There are no words to describe what that has meant to me ... unless they be: I Love You! Each and every one of you!!

III

Coming of Age, Generally: Well, each of us has our individual coming of age story to tell, each and every one of us thinks ours is unique. When viewed through a looking glass with a broader lens, however, there are maybe a handful of stories, all in a similar vein. My coming-of-age story is just one that our culture likes to frame as an ideal way to manhood – a story that involves one of our most revered national pastimes.

So, thank you football for your contribution to my coming-of-age story and all the character traits I've learned from that. However, I will discover that most of how I will deal with cancer will, of necessity, be learned day-to-day, as I go along.

It's often said that a person's coming-of-age story is the most important story of them all – the initial pathway chosen that then affects all the future ways we will walk on this earth. It's also said that a coming of age story can become parody, played out throughout one's lifetime – even though better stories would serve adults far better as they progressed through life.

And so, I wonder: has my story made me a prisoner to the cultural mores of my pubescent past; or has time and maturity worked to change what I really am? Has there been more inner change than just the drop of chest into Buddha-belly; more outer change than just the color of my hair, the withering of skin? Or have I been permanently wed to the me that existed at age-18, joyfully running pass routes?

I am convinced that most coming-of-age stories have a huge chunk of the Fates involved, perhaps along with the acquisition of a certain amount of skill and cunning that required the back-story of good coaching, and the wisdom of teachings from aged gurus … maybe coupled with a small smattering of grit, deter-mination, and persistence. My story is no exception.

IV

Last words: Oh yeah, about the coming-of-age story. Re-member that mine was more to impress my dad than to satisfy any of my own needs. Well, my dad died in a plane crash during my freshman year … and he never got to see me play even one minute of college ball.

Where does the impact of a storyline such as that hit the hard-est? To this day, I cannot point a finger to any specific body part … or to any one part of my spirit … or to any segment of my soul.

All I can say is that it certainly feels that I have held on to bits and pieces of the story – as it was writ through football – for a hell of a long time. Mostly, today I am seeing that tenacious grappling for holding on to the chest-thumping, fist-pumping, frog-croaking, flag-waving, team color-wearing caricature that included me as the resident tough guy … as one huge parody.

I guess the joke's on me.

But, of course, today I am no longer coming of age at 18; that was a good six decades ago – dinosaurs were still roaming the landscape. It's with the hint of nostalgia that I leave my carica-ture behind … and set out to write in my new character … with-out parody.

Perhaps, with a wee bit O' Me Irish Luck, I'll be able to use some of those skills I learned on the football gridiron … to help me play the game cancer has brought to me.

Chapter 13 Interlude: Football

I

Football: "Football instills important life lessons. Football is more than just a game; it teaches lessons that the players carry with them long after they've hung up their cleats" – this from people who study such things … and have absolutely no dog in the hunt.

The following are just a few of the lessons football teaches: teamwork, discipline, perseverance, goal-setting, handling success and failure, time management, keeping fit, and … and, um, in the several dozen scientific studies and popular media articles I reviewed, you can insert about any positive trait you can possibly dredge up from underneath a field of artificial turf … and insert it here_____.

In other words, football is, seemingly, the be-all and end-all, ultimate activity for developing a young man into the finest example of positive character traits that anyone could possibly imagine. Unless.

Unless you read the fine print. As someone who has been there, done that (on the collegiate gridiron at least), here's how the fine print reads to me (and I pick just a few examples):

Teamwork: Yes, football involves teamwork … but the teamwork of football – in order to select the final team that gets to play on Saturday – has been sifted through the finest mesh of competition one could imagine. If you don't kick the ass of anyone who plays at your position, he plays, and you sit.

Discipline and Goal Setting: Sure, there's a hell of a lot of discipline and goal setting going on around a football team. Problem is, it all comes down from the top, from the shouted exhortations of the coaches. Developing any internal discipline or learning how to set one's own goals is not a priority … and thus is something that needs to be learned after your football-playing days are over, if ever.

Time Management: Ha! If you mean that football will be your year-round, all-consuming activity for all the years you are playing, then I'd say that football *might* have something to do with teaching and developing the skills of time management.

Keeping Fit: Yep. You'd damned well better keep fit during and off season … or you will pay – extra laps, puking while doing warm ups, dying at the end of practice (or before). But, take a long look at the Buddha bellies of x-ballplayers, and then try to tell me that keeping fit has stuck with them after football.

Perseverance and Learning how to Accept Success and Failure: Football does indeed, in my opinion, teach these. And I would add one final one, a character trait you don't hear many of the folks involved in the Institutions of Sports talk about: pain tolerance.

Pain Tolerance: My grandsons all asked me if I thought they should play football. My answer was always: "Only if you like, really like, pain." I think, to play football and have fun playing it, you need to have more than just pain tolerance; you need to actually enjoy pain. Best answer I can give for acquiring this trait is to have it passed on to you, in your genes.

And so, as with most things, football's ability to enhance positive character traits is a mixed bag of do-goods, and do-nothings. Most of the do-goods are the result of having a demanding and effective coach. What you do after the coach leaves your life is left entirely up to you.

As I progress with my dance with cancer, I will need all I can get from the last three of the character traits listed above – perseverance (knowing that I need to stick with the treatment regime), knowing how to accept success and failure (some days will be good; others bad as hell); and pain tolerance (this one I'll need in excess).

Gurus

I

Introduction: Guru is a Sanskrit term for a "mentor, guide, expert, or master of a certain knowledge or field."

II

The Haunting of Gurus: It is already several months into my ACD (After Cancer Diagnosis) days, and I am struggling with how to write a memoir that is worth reading. I've gone through several iterations for how that task should be approached … when out of the blue a mentor from my deep dark past comes to mind. My guru-from-the-past was a fellow veterinarian named John Edward Lessin, but folks who knew him called him either "Jack" or "The Bear" – The Bear, an apt name for someone of his size and bearing.

I met The Bear while shopping for yet another job, an oft-repeated chore throughout my lifetime. This time I had chosen California as my next land of opportunity, and so had driven out there with hope in my heart.

By some stroke of good luck, I hooked up with the secretary of the California Veterinary Association who kept track of all the jobs currently available. One call later and I was headed north to Marin County, north of the San Francisco area where a group of veterinarians was forming a clinic to handle off-hours emergencies.

Dr. Lessin was the veterinarian in charge of hiring, and it didn't take long to learn that he was an Iowa State graduate who had, just as I had, played football there. Nor was it long before The Bear and I began our sessions of me being mentored by a bear.

Our sessions were typically held in the rec room of his huge house located at the cul-de-sac of a redwood-lined street in Larkspur that marked a major trail leading to the foot of Mount Tam.[12]

It was a dark room, a pool table in its midsection, off to one side a standup bar (stocked with plenty of beer), and a free-standing chalkboard that stood next to the bar. There was always music in the background – music too loud to my liking, but music still.

The chalkboard was the key to the room; the beer and pool table mere distractions. Scrawled across the board were words of wisdom, diagrams, arrows pointing in seemingly random directions, smudges of partially erased thoughts. The board was one of The Bear's ways of dealing with his world – his way of coming to grips.

I think, in his mind, I was there as one of the disciples, offering a tribute of sorts to his way of thinking. In my mind, the free beer was the key.

The scribblings in chalk, the conversations, the vibe – all of them mostly focused on one key problem with society as The Bear saw it: "Systems and Institutions of society were all initially created to serve mankind," he'd say. "All of them have, over time, transformed into institutions that mankind must now serve."

So, we'd talk about that, shoot some pool, have another beer, and when nature called, head outside to pee on the huge redwood tree that towered just outside the back door.

The Bear had a ritual when peeing. First, he'd extend hands and fingernails up onto the tree's enormous trunk and stretch and scratch. Then, when he'd finished peeing, he'd give a straight-arm shiver to the tree. Then, if we'd had enough beer, a forearm blast to the tree. Finally, he'd look skyward, up into the tree limbs, and say wistfully: "Well, that just proves it once again. Man will never be as good as a tree. We will never measure up to the powers of nature."

After watching his example for a while, I got to where I too could deliver a pretty good forearm blow to the tree – without hurting myself too much. Two x-football guys – thinking we still had it. Wasn't long before I could see beyond the macho

---

12 Mt Tam to locals; Mount Tamalpais to visitors. Mt Tam is a 2,500-foot high mountain in Marin County where, from its peak, you have a 360° view from San Francisco Bay to the Pacific. Nature is everywhere on "Tam." Miles and miles of trails ribbon the mountain, crossing redwood valleys, creeks, waterfalls, and wide-open grasslands. It has been treasured turf for hikers, cyclists, and equestrians since the 1880s.

and feel the honor of belief in nature as the ultimate source of wisdom and healing ... all this without even once hugging that huge redwood.

One day, I was curious about the background music which always seemed to sound the same. It was music I kinda liked but not my favorite sound, which trended more toward Johnny Cash. So, I asked The Bear: "Who is that singing?"

He looked at me astonished: "You mean you don't know?" Jack asked, incredulous. "You really don't know?" "Yeah," I said. "I'm not much of a music man."

"Well, that's Janice Joplin," replied The Bear. "This was once her house. She was a client of mine with her pets, and she and I had long conversations – me trying to get her to think in bigger terms, to ask what the institutions were doing to her (instead of for her), to think in terms of nature as the ultimate teacher. I think I almost had her thinking that way too ... when she took her life."

"After she died," Jack continued, "her entourage came to me and said they couldn't think of anyone else who they would feel comfortable living in her house. Would I please buy it? And so I did, and here we are."

III

Last Words: Jack "The Bear" Lessin: guru to a rock and roll icon ... and to a hillbilly from Ohio (via Iowa) who now can write a memoir on Walking in Nature with Cancer with four main themes:

1. Institutions (for example: medicine, and especially oncology) are initially developed to serve mankind; those institutions eventually become entangling webs that mankind is forced to serve.
2. There is no better healer nor teacher than Nature.
3. Stop, look and learn, listen and feel, respect.
4. It pays to listen to the background music and to ask questions about what it might mean.

Chapter 14 Interlude: Gurus Galore

I

Gurus Galore: I am convinced that gurus are sent to each and every one of us … from some strange place that will remain forever unknown. (You can call them gurus or any number of other names, including: mentors, teachers, instructors, guides, coaches, parents, etc., but I personally like the term "guru" for the dark and hidden truths it conjures.)

I have the sense that a true guru appears without your asking for one: out of the blue you suddenly are confronted by someone who has something of profound interest and wisdom to offer. It then becomes your choice as to whether or not to accept the offerings … or to go on your merry old way.

As a participant in the guru-ing, you need to listen intently, ask questions, analyze and respect the answers, and take some form of action. That's it. At least I think those are the rules. What I can tell you with certainty is that I never planned for, hoped for, asked for, nor prayed for any of the gurus who came my way – again from some unknown place. And boy howdy, I've been mentored by some of the best gurus on earth – just by paying attention ... a trait you learn from Nature.

II

Seven Generations: There's one final thing about guru-ing I think is important. I'm convinced that we are, each of us, sent here to be a guru/mentor/teacher/ coach/etc. for someone else. I see this as a part of the Native American concept of Seven Generations whereby each generation is beholden to the teachings of the three previous generations and is also responsible for the caretaking and teaching of those three generations that follow.

The final requisite in the Seven Generations concept is that the present generation (ours) is responsible for determining what it is that the Great Spirit wants us to do during our lifetime. That is, we are responsible for figuring out why we are here … and for doing something positive with that recognition.

III

Family of Gurus: At 80+ years of age, I'm still working on that last part of the Seven Generations thingy – a tribute to how quick a learner I am. But here's how it seems to be working out for me:

1. I have been blessed with mentoring from both parents and grandparents – blessed far beyond any possible expectation. I didn't know any of my great-grandparents, but I have a lot to be thankful for, given to me via my Irish genes. For example: my hard-headedness, pain tolerance, Irish sense of joie de vivre with its moderating sense of melancholia … all this along with the cancer-enhancing genes I carry with me.

2. I could not have dreamed of a better guru for showing me how to live than my Sue. She has always been my rock, my confidence builder and chief supporter, my example of how to actually live a life of joy … and now my cancer caretaker who always seems to know when to crack the whip, when to cajole, and when to offer sympathy.

3. Sue and I tried to be good parents, good mentors for those life-ways we thought important. But what has happened is that, over the years, our three daughters (along with their spouses) have become our prime life-time gurus – each of them contributing her own personality to the task of mentoring us old folks, and each of them now showing us how we should have been living all along.

4. In addition, each of these three daughters had children (our grandchildren) who have now become our life gurus – giving us, with their subtly supplied examples, clues for how we *should* be living our lives.

5. And then the great grandchildren started coming along, our little bundles of joy. What a joy: watching them as they grow up … and as they are in turn mentored by their parents and grandparents – without Sue and I having to lift a finger.

IV

Last Words: And so, through all the Seven Generations, the circle of Sue's and my life has remained unbroken ... thanks at least in part to the presence of all those gurus who appeared out of nowhere to offer us wisdom, advice, encouragement, challenge, and support.

I can hear Johnny Cash's gravely voice now, just a-singin' it to the rafters on high:

Will the circle be unbroken
By and by, Lord, by and by?
There's a better home awaiting
In the sky, Lord, in the sky.

Animal Gurus

I

Mountain Horses: Grandpa on Dad's side stuck with the farming skills he'd learned as a kid, and he continued to use many of the same skills our kinfolk brought over from Ireland. He was heir to the farm his great grandfather had settled on in the early 1800s – about 100 acres of mostly pasture with a few cropland fields and a small patch of woodland hidden behind the back forty.

Grandpa brought with him a work ethic that had him working in a series of full time jobs in the dairy industry and in various other jobs located in nearby Columbus – the farming he did was part-time, after work. In those hours he was able to run a small herd of Hereford cattle, milk a few cows, help with the annual farrowing of several litters of piglets, and watch over a flock of free-range chickens.

Plus – and this was a biggie plus for the growing-up me – he worked a huge "truck" garden with a team of horses; horses I called "Grandpa's Mountain Horses" ... because that's what they looked like to three-foot-tall me. Grandpa seemed to really enjoy the chance to throw us grandkids up on the back of one of those horses. And I loved being up there – me with my legs sprawled almost straight out over horse ribs, and hanging on to horse mane for dear life.

From the top of a Mountain Horse, I loved the warmth of just-worked horse flesh, the steady in and out heave of equine breathing, the smell of sweaty horse hair, the feeling of what to my young heart was like being on top of all the power in the world.

They say that for many people the smell of chocolate chip cookies baking in the oven activates primitive brain areas that remind you of the good feelings you developed long ago while visiting Grandma. So sure, I like the smell of chocolate chip cookies baking, but if I really want to feel good all over, I'll walk into a horse barn.

The smell of horse and horse sweat, mixed with aroma of hay and straw along with added hints of horse breath; and the final odorific punctuation of horse shit and horse piss are enough to bring back great memories of both Grandma and Grandpa

– but also the cherished memories of those many hours I've spent alongside horses, learning good horse sense from them.

II

Polar Bear: So, memories from childhood some seven decades past can have profound effects, and it is said that your first memories often hold special places in the development of your later-on self.

Several years back, my mom and I were reminiscing on our pasts and I mentioned the time we were at a zoo, watching the antics of a polar bear. This was back before we realized that feeding the animals junk food was probably not good for them, and I remember my dad had a box of popcorn for us to munch on. For some reason, he flipped the box over the fence into the polar bear's pen, and the bear immediately grabbed it and buried his snout deep into the box. Then he sat up, leaned back, and shook that box until he'd swallowed the last of the crumbs.

I remember I must have thought that was the most comical thing I'd ever seen, and I laughed gleefully, as only a child can do. It is very likely, at that age, I also peed my pants … but I don't remember that part of the story.

Anyway, when I related this story, my mom said, "You remember that? Why Randy, you couldn't have been more than two years old. That would have been the Dallas Zoo, and we went there while we were still stationed at Randolph Field."

So this, one of the first etchings on a young lad's mind, comes from an animal.

III

Freckles: I am in first or second grade. By then I'd had a long list of pets, but my dad, being a country boy, never let the dogs sleep in the human quarters. Freckles was special, a Dalmatian that earned the privilege of sleeping in the unattached garage … I think because she was pregnant. She whelped a litter of nine pups out there, and I was, of course, fascinated. I spent many long hours, out in our garage, watching over mother and her brood.

My mom, not a big keeper of memorabilia, for some reason kept a particular scribbling of mine, related to Freckles. It was only a few lines scrawled on a huge sheet of paper … but they were profound. And, the accompanying art work had – at least in my family's thoughts – a sense of depth akin to Andy Warhol's soup can art.

I'm thinking that early aspirations for me, coming from my family, were related to my becoming a writer or perhaps an artist … not necessarily working with animals. In fact, when I told my dad I wanted to be a veterinarian, he reminded me – time and time again – "Look Randy, if you become a doctor, a *real* doctor, you can own all the damned animals you'd ever want."

Fooled them all, didn't I?

IV

Hard Lessons: I don't know how old I was, but probably old enough to know better. I got tired of adult talk around Grandpa and Grandma's huge round dinner table, so I slipped away to go see the Mountain Horse's new foal – just a few weeks old.

Momma and foal had a huge stall to themselves, and to my young senses the whole barn had taken on the smell of newness. It was an old-style barn with dirt floors and the double stall where mom and babe were staying was separated from the aisle by a feed and hay manger, with double walls about four feet high and the manger part some three feet across.

It was about all I could do to climb into the manger, then crawl out the other side – into the stall with those two I wanted to see up close and personal. Fortunately, very fortunately, the mare was lying down; she took one look at me as I crawled into the stall, sighed, and laid her head back down. Colt had jumped up at my arrival, but he too looked to mom and then laid back down beside her.

It was the perfect place for a young lad to prop his little body up against the mare's back and dream about working with horses … as I watched the colt – who was already shut-eyed and breathing into his own dreams. I remember melting into the rhythm of mare breathing when I heard them calling for me. Their calls woke momma and she very carefully got up, walked over to the outside doorway, stuck her head out the opened half of the doorway, and neighed that she knew where I was.

When they found me, I got read the riot act by both Grandpa and Dad – yeah verily, once again. I did avoid the trip to behind the woodshed … but barely. "Son, don't you know that horses can be dangerous. They can kill you with one flick of hoof. Don't you ever do that again. Ever!"

As I say: I was lucky. Damned lucky. But my oh my, what a memory I carry with me … to this very day.

V

More Lessons: There are other lessons, of course; lessons you should be old enough that they shouldn't need to be taught. Many of those. Take for example the time I caught a nice little garter snake sunning on a limb down in the woods behind our house. Caught him clean (after screwing up my courage for an hour or more) and had him in a death grip so I could take him home to show mom.

Well, the death grip failed, he worked his head loose, and the little bastard bit me. Snap. Snap. Snap. Three times. His bites felt like being "bit" by someone pressing a tiny stickle burr into your skin – no fangs nor fang marks involved here. Yes, I know garter snakes are supposed to be non-poisonous, so no big deal, right? But almost immediately upon being bitten by the non-poisonous snake, I got the chills, my hands started shaking, and I had to stop walking and catch my breath. And, of course, I dropped the snake. I still don't know if I was simply having the adrenalin-induced fear response, or did the little shit deposit enough poison into my body to cause the reaction.

In any event, you learn about the nuances of Nature … by having living experiences with them. This includes, of course, the experience of being attacked by chiggers, ticks, mosquitoes, bees, wasps, and so on. And dealing with poison ivy, stinging nettles, and sticky burrs. And having the weather not give a damn about your plans for the day. And on and on. So be it.

VI

Last Words: I actually like the challenges of being in Nature. And I've always felt more comfortable around animals (wild and tame) than I've ever felt when being around the human animal. I take both solace and challenge from being in Nature ... in association with the animals that have become my gurus.

Finally, I realize this kinship feeling with nature and especially animals may not be the norm for the current place my species has put itself in. I realize that most people would prefer being around other people. And I get it that some people feel comfortable in large crowds and are seemingly made to feel even more comfortable (or is it more powerful) by yelling across the room at each other. Just not my cup of tea.

Give me some of that stinging nettle (or mullein, or sassafras) tea instead. And let me be in the quiet of Nature somewhere, preferably in the company of some wild animal species.

Chapter 15 Interlude:
Ho Mitakuye Oyasin

I

At First Sweat: I have a friend who, during his annual physical, discovered he had an elevated PSA (prostate-specific antigen). Not too bad for his age, but something to be concerned about enough that he should keep track of it. And so, he asked me if he could go with me to an inipi (sweat lodge purification ceremony) to see if that would help.

I checked with some friends with local Native American connections; they helped set it up for us; and there we were along with another dozen or so half-naked celebrants entering the lodge and repeating: "Ho Mitakuye Oyasin" as we entered and then again as we exited.

This was not the first-time inipi for me, but it was for my friend. When we had left the heat of the lodge and were out into the cool of night, getting back into our clothes, he pulled me aside and asked: "So, what's that stuff they say when going in and out? What's that all about?"

"Oh, yeah," I said, "'Mitakuye Oyasin,' means something like, 'All my relations.' It's a prayer of sorts."

"All my relations, eh," he says. "Hell's fire, I can't stand most of my relations. My family is, and always has been, one big screwed up mess."

And so, I try to explain that it's not just your family that you are honoring; it's your connection to all beings, your interconnection to everything in the universe – animal, vegetable, mineral … and not just to your human family, but also to the entire family of humans."

And my friend says, "Oh, well that makes a huge difference. So, Ho Mitakuye Oyasin to you, my friend."

II

Mitakuye Oyasin: is a phrase from the Lakota language that translates to "all my relatives," "we are all related," or "all my relations." It is a prayer of oneness and harmony with all forms of life: other people, animals, birds, insects, trees and plants, and even rocks, rivers, mountains and valleys.

The phrase reflects the Lakota world view of the interconnectedness of all things and is often expressed in prayers or as part of Lakota ceremonies. I often think of Mitakuye Oyasin as a phrase that opens my awareness to the constant presence of Nature's many interconnections I am thankful for.

III

Thanks Be: There's so much to be thankful for: Every day it all starts with the rising sun – I am alive for yet another day. Sue and I have our traditional brekker of: sliced avocado (thank you avocado tree) and tomatoes (thank you tomato plants) over multi-seed toast (thank you to a whole realm of seed plants, yeast, and whole-wheat flour), all this topped off with a poached egg (thank you chickens). And then there's the coffee and the maple syrup I use for sweetener and the yogurt and kefir I sip on – more thanks to the maple trees and the coffee bean bushes and the milk cows and to whatever little bugs were used to fester the milk into healthy probiotics.

And thanks to all the humans that brought those plants (and eggs and milk) to us. And thanks for the salt and pepper and ground turmeric I use for flavoring and medicinal value.

And thanks for the web that maintains all of this as a huge interconnection to the pollinator critters and to the winds and waters that keep the plants alive. And thanks to the interconnections between the insects and the birds … and us.

And thanks to the dirt of the earth itself and for all that's within that dirt – the wee crawly-creatures, the fungi, and the roots of plants … all of those that give sustenance to the plants growing above. And thanks to the Earth Mother Herself for providing the Nature and Nurture that sustains us all.

And an astronomic thank you to the stars above for giving us the stardust we are all made from – each and every one of us, whether we be animal, vegetable or mineral … or some combination of all three.

And thanks to … well, you get the idea. Trying to give all the Ho Mitakuye Oyasins the earth deserves can be exhausting.

IV

Last Words: Sue and I usually sit at the brekker table and reminisce about our family and the friends (and the not-so-friendly folks) we have met along the way – their stories make us laugh (and sometimes cry). This sojourn-of-sorts sets the tone for the rest of the day: a day that will hopefully get me out and about in Nature – where I can interconnect with all that She brings to this new day. And hopefully it will be another day that will give me the opportunity to write a few more words into my memoir.

So much to be thankful for. So much positive has happened since the universe decided to drop some rogue cancer cells into my system. So many "Ho Mitakuye Oyasins" to say. Each and every day.

And by the way, my friend with the elevated PSA? Well, it's been at least a decade, maybe more like two decades ago when we were in the inipi together … and he tells me his PSA has stayed the same since way back then. Plus, he has never had any of the symptoms of prostate cancer.

Family Kidd Plus

I

Opening Stage Setting: The kitchen area of a third floor apartment. Stage left is the dining area with four chairs surrounding the antique-wood dining table (each chair a different style, color, and vintage). Further stage left is the living room with sofa, easy chair, and rocker, all placed for easy viewing of the TV on the wall. Hidden from view, stage left, is the spare bedroom (Randy's office) and the bathroom.

Stage right is the kitchen – stove, refrigerator, sink and plenty of counter space with cupboards along the wall. There is a large C-shaped island in the middle of the kitchen – a water filter and potted plant at one end and a bowl of various fruits at the other. Prominently placed in the island's middle is a photo screen that continuously runs images of family members and their activities.

Further Stage Right and out of sight are the master bedroom and bathroom.

II

Act 1: Our two actors, Sue and Randy Kidd, are sitting on barstools facing the kitchen island's photo screen. We learn that the barstools were gifts from their grown children … after the children learned that the original pair had been lifted from a dumpster by Sue, she of exquisite dumpster-diving skills. We also learn that the photo screen was provided by the children – as was a figure known as Alexa who apparently lives on top of an antique sewing-machine converted to a small table that sits next to the dining room table, as was the dining room and kitchen light-fixtures … because the children thought the initial ones were far too outdated.

Sue and Randy are glued intently to the photo screen, gesticulating, telling stories, whooping and hollering … and sometimes even crying. The screen is a treasure chest of recent memories – memories of family and friends. Sue gets up every few minutes to check and stir the cut-up brats she has browning on the stove, waiting until just the right moment to add-in their favorite locally-made kraut.

We learn that this or some rendition of it is a good part of the story of how Sue and Randy are living out their final years. Were we to spend a day with them we would listen as they talked – over the dining room table – of the family haps, both current and from years ago.

After brekker, Sue would be busy, busy, busy … with gardening chores, the task of being a Board Member of our Village Co-op, getting her daily walking-miles in, going to Physical Therapy or Rolfing sessions … and being a caretaker for Randy. Randy too would be busy, busy – trying to put words together for his memoir, walking in nature, and napping.

Lunchtime would be more storytelling, as with dinner. You get the idea: stories of family, of family outings, and family events – all shared and relayed by photo or storytelling; stories of family successes and failures and of family trials and tribulations … and the stories of how the family members handled all of these.

Play-acting this storyline could be thought of as a reflection of Shakespeare's seven stages of life: infancy, schoolboy, teenager, young man, middle age, old age, and death. All these (save for the last one) have been lived by the Kidds; they are now able to relive them through their family members, as those family members are moving through them.

But for the Kidds, the stories of family are just there – there to reflect the importance of family as a part of life.

Underlying all this is the ominous presence of Randy's cancer, fogging up the inner and outer landscape … and requiring a presence of focus and determination to adequately deal with the vagaries of the disease, and to deal with end of life planning.

It's been said that it takes a family to raise a child; it also takes a family to help someone walk that final, end-of-life, walk.

III

Act Two: The changing of background scenery will take us on a tour of Sue and Randy's humble abode. Each scenery change will transport us into another room, the room's walls almost covered with framed photos. Along the living room's huge wall is a collection of animal art, each drawn by someone Sue and Randy knew … and so each one containing, within the boundaries of its framework, a story or two.

A corner wall in the master bedroom is devoted to photos of their three daughters as they were growing up … and then as they gained their spouses and children. Another wall in that room is filled with grandchildren, and a final bedroom wall – the "wedding wall" – is devoted to the grandchildren and their spouses as they were married.

There is a small hallway leading into the kitchen and on one side are photos of Sue and Randy's parents and grandparents. In a niche space along the other wall is a photo-shelf, hand-tooled by one of the grandchildren, that is crammed with photos of great-grandchildren and their parents. Hidden among these pictures is one of a young Randy atop one of his "mountain horses;" – Grandpa Kidd with a huge smile, holding onto the reins.

Mixed in with all these photos are others of Sue and Randy's extended families – spouses of their children and grandchildren and then of their families; and also those many folks the Kidds have gotten to know so well that they are considered family. And now the folks of the cooperative Village – all of these folks are also a part of the Kidd's Big Family.

Put this huge family together and Sue and Randy have been gifted with countless stories to tell and to reminisce over.

Scattered hither and thither throughout the apartment are artworks painted by family, rocks and plants collected from nature, animal figurines and fetishes – stuff collected along the way that are now referred to as "memorabilia." Finally, for the great-grandkids to play with, a basket full of critter puppets, and standing in a corner, a floppy-eared stuffed black dog named Buddy.

Act two is a mélange of stories, each prompted by a photo on the wall or one of the pieces of memorabilia. Many of the stories are of what's happening to a particular family member today – information that has come via a recent phone call or a text (often with photos) from that member.

We know, for example, that a granddaughter has a new job, after being laid off from another a month or so ago. We know that there are two new puppies in two different families, and the Kidds now have videos of new-puppy antics.

To be honest, this act can become a mite sappy …unless you have a family of your own.

IV

Act Three: We see by a clock on the wall that it is about 8:00 pm; Sue and Randy are watching TV … or trying to. Both are having trouble keeping their eyes open, trying to steady their nodding of heads. We see one of them snap awake, wipe off the spot of spittle that's slowly drooling down their chin. They turn the TV off, get up, and head to a small outside deck at the southwest corner of their apartment. They take seat cushions with them, get set up on the metal porch chairs, and look to the skies.

They are there for the final stories, nighttime stories of how their days went; of what they expect for tomorrow; perhaps a story or two remembering something funny (or painful) about some family member. They have about an hour of coherence left in them … before they will get up and stagger back to bed.

V

Last Words: Sue and Randy are highly skilled star watchers. Together they can possibly name two or three stars or constellations from their deck – Orion the Hunter, the Seven Sisters. Maybe Venus.

But still, they look to the skies. And you hope they are able to let the audience in on a secret they know: that the Kidds, and everyone else in the Earth Family of humans, animals, vegetables, and minerals is a product of stardust … and all of us will ultimately return to that stardust.

Chapter 16 Interlude: Honeycomb

I

Background: We have in our Village family a couple that has recently remarried. One of them calls the other "Honey," which, when I heard it, I thought it was just the sweetest thing for one doddering old man to use as the name he called his baby. So, I – another doddering old-guy – started to call Sue "Honey," … which she loved.

Then, I remembered that 60-odd years ago, when I was courting Sue, for some strange reason, I took to serenading her with the then-popular song: Honeycomb. Once again, I'm sure she loved it. And so, I looked the lyrics up … and they apply perfectly (even if they might be a bit mushy) to my current feelings for her.

One evening, at the dinner table, as a surprise for my honey, I had Alexa play the song for us. Sue rolled her eyes – apparently in a joyful moment of rapture. And so, here are the lyrics. Hopefully your honey will have a similar response to how mine reacted.

II

"… Well it's a darn good life"

"Honeycomb" —Song by Jimmie Rodgers (and I think several others)

PART FOUR:
Stop;
Look, Listen, and Learn;
Respect

Walking in Nature

I

Thin Places: "Heaven and Earth," the Celtic saying goes, "are only three feet apart, but in thin places that distance is even shorter." An Apache proverb pushes this thought one step further: "Wisdom sits in places," they say.

Thin places are where heaven and earth collapse and we're able to catch glimpses of the divine, or the transcendent. Thin places are the sanctuaries where we bring ourselves to reunite our spirit with the soul of Nature. To the ancient pagan Celts and later Christians, thin places included mesmerizing settings like the wind-swept isle of Iona (now part of Scotland) or the rocky peaks of Croagh Patrick.

Typically, a thin place is like that: a high peak or an area of beauty where the cycles and the winds of nature prevail. But your personal thin places can occur anywhere: perhaps a favorite temple or church that offers a personal invitation to prayer. Or atop a lonely hillock on a tallgrass Kansas prairie where, as you are walking, the Big Bluestem grasses rattle their seeds overhead and where the winds undulate the grasses into a sea of waves. Or a quiet pub with hand-hewn backbar and chiseled beams overhead, where the beer is always cold and the conversation quiet and warm. Or that special place in the woods with its oaken, moss-covered windfall as the perfect place to sit and re-compose.

In short, a thin place can be anywhere that inspires, calms, and/or excites our inner Beings; any place that connects us with The Other; any place that enhances our lives and transforms us into our essential selves.

II

Walking in Nature: It is early March, 2019, about nine months after my surgery and nine months into chemotherapy. I feel almost fully gestated into the new me. I walk, now with the aid of my hiking sticks. Daily, I walk – except on those days when the chemo poisons have turned me into a sniveling, pitiful wimp, curled up on the couch.

I walk – sometimes I need to force myself to walk – because walking is my gateway to, and my prescription for, staying alive. I walk in Nature – in the nature provided me along city streets – because Nature is the ultimate healer. My ultimate healer. I walk along city sidewalks because I trip and stumble on uneven grounds; whereas I once was able to run right through the grasp of a mean-ass linebacker, now a tuft of grass can trip me up.

My daily walks are out the back door and onto sidewalks that take me on a one to two-mile round trip – all in all this gives me a fair look at a circle of suburban nature about a mile in radius.

In that circle of nature there's the empty field nearby where ruts of the Oregon Trail are still visible and where a family of redtail hawks and at least one fox family all live. There's the cut into the layers of limestone alongside Wakarusa Drive where a hibernaculum of black rat snakes spends the winter. There's a small forest of cedars where you can walk the gravel trail and almost feel the scent of cedar easing your mind; and there's our own Village swale – a detention pond packed with native plants that attract a host of birds and butterflies.

The awe-inspiring grandeur of nature can creep up on you and come at you from some very strange and odd-ball places; from directions unexpected. Within my walking circles there are two retention ponds that offer special looks at suburbanized nature.

III

Nature Highlights: My normal walking routes take me by a couple of retention ponds that hold some interest, one behind a MegaMart and the other between the Theatre Lawrence and Free State High School. The interest is in the nature they contain within, nature walled off from direct human intrusion by a surrounding iron fence that is fortified with several **NO TRES-PASSING** signs. Fittingly, I name my "Nature Centers:" Pond 1 and Pond 2.

The pond parts of my Nature Centers are dugouts, perhaps 30 feet below the sidewalks. Each pond is roughly the size of a football field, stretched and convoluted to fit into the curves of the landscape. Pond 1 is surrounded by rather steep fields of grasslands, climbing up from pond to fence. Pond 2 is situated inside surrounding stone walls, with small bits of sod and cattail marshland rimming the pond.

Both ponds represent a natural (sort of) wetlands, each with enough retained wet runoff to foster a thicket of cattails and other swampland plants: grasses and weeds, a few early-growth cottonwoods and willows, and a smattering of cedar trees.

Over the past few years I have watched ice and snow form and melt away over the course of the winter months, and I've been mesmerized on warmer days by the wind-driven undulations on the top of the ponds and across the seas of browned grasses.

My ponds have become my stop-and-meditate places; sites to breathe deeply and to relax my mind and my knees. Places to listen for the silent and not-so-silent sounds of nature; resting places to renew soul connections.

I have watched as the summers turn grey to green, and in each of the ponds I have spotted families of muskrats, going about their daily grind without paying me any heed.

Springtime mom and pop muskrat are busy as beavers, trotting up the hill to gnaw off tufts of grass, trotting back down with a mouthful of green, then swimming across the pond to their den's entrance where, depending on the family, they disappear under the shoreline or into their lodge made of cattail leaves. One summer I watched at least three baby kits playing on and around their lodge.

As I watch, I know there are many unseen wild eyes watching me in return. But, on occasion, in the depths of summer, there will be one set of eyes, sitting astride the serpentine snout of an ancient being. The eyes and beaked-snout will be poking up just above the water, keeping track of me. These are the eyes and nose of a rather nice sized snapping turtle, and if you look through binoculars, you can make out beneath the waters her shelled body and scaley-skinned legs.

Snapping turtles have been around for more than 70 million years. They lived with the dinosaurs, which means they survived the mass extinction that wiped the dinosaurs off the earth some 65 million years ago.

I am too far away to see this, but, were I nose-to-nose, toes-to-toes with her, and if I looked into her eyes, I would see eyes literally aglow with spark: deep black holes of pupils, surrounded by an iris of chicken-fat yellow. And then the spark of eye – a sky dotted with several black star-like dots, the dots connected inwardly to form a black cross or outwardly to resemble a starburst.

The eyes of a prehistoric being, watching this aging human being … watch her. Snapping turtles, to my way of thinking, offer physical evidence that most places in nature are really thin connections between heaven and earth.

IV

Retention Ponds: Admittedly a retention pond (think of what type of effluent it is detaining) is not particularly awe-inspiring. By mid-summer the area retention ponds will likely become festering, odoriferous puddles of green algae and muck; puddles inundated with wind-blown trash; and "wetlands" where noxious weeds will be the main crop – hardly a place where one's first thought is: "this sure feels like it's a thin place."

Sue refuses to stand with me in the summertime as I watch over my ponds and the nature within. She says, "It stinks too bad down there – and look at all that trash." But my ponds are *my* thin places – no matter (to me) that they come with a healthy dose of grunge and grit.

V

Looking Deeper: But if you can think deep enough, if you can imagine the physicality of my ponds – deep within the fenced-in areas – as entrances to the underground earth, you might be able to imagine the tall grasses and trees as growths on a pelvic girdle; the muddy shoreline as labia, lip-like connections where water and ground opens into the womb of the earth.

Even with all the evidence of human intrusion, for me it is not difficult to see the Nature within. For me, the overwhelming feel of my retention ponds as thin places always prevails – two common places along my walking trails where the divine meets with Me, The Mundane.

But this is March, and I have yet to be treated to the main attraction: the migration of birds that will arrive along with the warming sun. There will be both seed and bug-eater birds: red winged blackbirds will chatter from the cattails, swallows will swoop and scoop bugs from the water surface, and at Pond 1 there will be at least two families of bug-catching Eastern King-birds that will take up summertime residence in the cottonwoods.

VI

Last Words: The biggest attraction, however, the part of nature that will hold my fascination for most of that first summer (and for several summers to come), will be bird families that have the ability to transport me away from my thoughts of the inevitability of death and dying … into the realm of new birth, regeneration, and further appreciation for the creatures of nature.

It's early spring and my families of geese have not yet flown in. But they will, and I will soon be talking with them. I will become a part of their families and I will rejoice with them their accomplishments … and suffer with them their heartaches.

Interlude Chapter 17: Synanthropes

Synanthropes: A synanthrope is a member of a species of wild animal or plant that lives near, and benefits from, an association with humans and the artificial habitats that these beings have created.

Well, I'll be damned. All those critters and plants that I've been communing with, searching for a deeper meaning through Nature – all of them are synanthropic. (I can't wait to use the term at our next men's coffee klatch.)

Now I can look that varmint squirrel in the eye – he the squirrel who adores the oaks that have been planted as backyard landscape trees, and he the rodent wizard who cannot be kept out of the bird feeders – and say to his face: "Lookee here nutty buddy. You're nothing more than a synanthrope."

I can say the same thing to the crows who run a scouting party on our garbage bins every day. And to the raccoons and possums who, when you put the dog's dish outside the backdoor, will be there within minutes with their feasting bibs already tied on.

"You're nothing more than synanthropes," I can shout out at the dandelions that have festered our lawn, and at the cottonwood trees that line the creek beds and ponds, and the ... well, you get the idea.

Pretty much everything I see on my walks through the city are synanthropes – living beings that have learned how to take advantage of the spoils of humanity. And I say: "More power to them."

II

Goose Whiners: I've already mentioned that the geese that inhabit my Ponds are one of my favorite spirits of nature. On the other hand, I'm sure there are people out there who don't love Canada geese. "They crap on the sidewalks," they whine – forgetting that they, the whiners, also crap ... and then flush their own crap into the waterways that support all life. 'Tis true that crap is stinky, slippery stuff, but 'tis also true that, if treated right, it is biodegradable into a fertile addendum to field and garden.[13]

'Tis furthermore true that human crap contains the toxins and poisons (including chemo-therapy poisons), plastics and detergents, and (perhaps worst of all) the residues of antibiotics and opioids that the crapper has ingested. But the goose didn't

---

13 For a time there we raised domestic geese, and I have felt their wrath first hand. One day in particular I was working in the barn where the geese stayed, and I had just squatted down to pick up a feeder. From out of nowhere, I got waylaid by a forearm shiver delivered by the leading edge of an extended goose wing. Hit me square on the bridge of my nose, buckled my legs, and I saw stars for a long time afterward. This from a 15 to 20 pound angry goose; not a 250 pound angry linebacker.

invent all the crap that goes into our human crap, and isn't it true that we should be blaming ourselves for contaminating our waters with our own crap? The grass and weed-eating goose is only an innocent bystander to the damages we have brought to ourselves.

'Tis also true that Canada geese can be fierce defenders of their turf and especially of their clan – they can easily whoop up on most dogs who want to chase, and kids are often terrified of them.[14]

In Canada recently, a visitor who was being harassed by a Canada goose protecting her brood, referred to her as that "Hissing Cobra Chicken" … a name that has, for me at least, stuck. (T-shirts with the Hissing Cobra Chicken standing proudly, wings outstretched, under the Canadian flag are available on the internet.)

III

The Demise of the Ponds: This year, both families of geese disappeared when the little ones were about a month old – far too early for them to be able to fend for themselves or fly away. Word on the street was that "The City" removed them – they were too much bother and people were complaining. Damned synanthropes.

And here's what happened after they disappeared: the ponds died. At least the crappy stink that arose out of the ponds told us the story: Death has arrived. A green scum quickly blanketed the ponds' surfaces, and once-clear water turned mucky murkey.

Worst of all (for me the Nature watcher): All non-scum life left the ponds. The swallows that had nested in the inlet and outlet culverts disappeared, robins and sparrows and Eastern and Western Kingbirds also gone. The herons – Great and Little Blue, and Green – stopped dropping by for an occasional fish or bullfrog dinner. There were no more eyes of bullfrog nor snapping turtle watching me. The sounds of Nature had gone silent.

---

14 And by the way: I'd like to see a fair fight between any dog of the same weight as the goose – a typical wild goose will weigh about 5 to 14 pounds, with some scaling up to about 20 pounds. Thus the fight would be between goose and Chihuahua or, at the upper end of the scale between goose and Lhasa Apso or Shih tzu, or Miniature Poodle.

The rapid demise of the ponds, without geese, makes you think that, instead of being problem children, the geese may truly be the keystone species of the ponds. (**Keystone species:** a species on which other species in an ecosystem largely depend, such that if it were removed, the ecosystem would change drastically.)

And so, as always, Nature has its Yin/Yang; has its nuances. I'm convinced we humans will never be able to settle our differences ... until and unless we respect all beings around us as if they were a part of our family. Furthermore, we need to quit bellyaching about all our supposed pains and injuries; we need to take responsibility for the pains and the injuries we cause ourselves. End of lecture.

IV

Last Words: Finally, it seems to me that we are the true and original synanthropes. It is we who have clumped together in order to take advantage of our associations with other humans and to sop up the spoils from the artificial habitats those same humans have created.

Welcome to the club, fellow synanthrope.

Spirit of Hawk

I

Introduction: Sometimes, when things look their bleakest, a messenger comes along and soars into your heart, breathes light into your soul, and sets the tone of spirit that will carry you through the rest of the day ... or the rest of your life. Lately, hawks have been the most persistent presence in my life; messengers from above.

II

Hawk: Hawk has long been a friend of mine, a friendship that began in veterinary school, way back when. A fellow veterinary student in my class was a falconer. Jim, who has since become a veterinary surgeon of some renown, always had one bird he was working with, and while we were in school, he typically kept his current bird tethered to the foot of the bed he shared with his wife.

While we were still vet students, Jim took me out to watch one of his bird's early flights. This was a Red-tailed hawk he had worked with for some time – teaching her to come to his out-stretched arm for food. He warned me that the bird, seeing it was free, might not return.

"In fact," he said, "that's what happens most of the time." And so, he released the bird, she flew out away from us, then began an ascent, climbing in circles up, up, and away, catching the Iowa wind, soaring higher and higher until she was a speck in the sky. And then I lost her. She was gone.

But I wasn't the seasoned hawk-watcher Jim was. I followed his pointing finger, and there she was: a blur of silver catching the sunlight, a feathered rocket coming straight down, an incredible display of what a hawk's stoop looks like. Then, she was gone again – her dive taking her to the other side of a small rise in the prairie. Jim's face said it all: She wanted freedom more than she needed human companionship.

Then, from nowhere, she came out of some indentation in the grasses, took three wingstrokes directly toward us, swooped up from ground level, and landed gracefully on Jim's outstretched and gloved arm. Mission accomplished.

That bit of falconry happened more than five decades ago, and I can still see the hawk's glint of eyes and her outstretched wings as she came straight at us. Is it any wonder, then, that I look for hawks wherever I go? Any wonder that when I see one, out of respect, I nod and send a silent "Ho Mitakuye Oyasin" their way.

III

The Trespassers: It's springtime 2018, and there we are: three old-folk couples, three stories high, looking out onto the deck that Sue and I will eventually be sitting on. We are trespassing, checking the progress being made (if any) on our home-to-be, an apartment unit in the southwest corner, third floor of a 52-unit cooperative complex.

The Co-op is called The Village, and it will eventually house us as we age into senility. Already the builders are more than 18 months behind schedule, and they are acting as if that's normal, as if it's normal to make a host of people who are looking forward to spending their last years in the comfort of a community of like-minded, like-aged folks sit on their thumbs for what could be the last 18 months of their lives.

We are there with the trepidation of the law breaker, with the helpless fury of those who have been stepped upon, lied to, and treated as pawns by BigCon (Big Construction), and with the hope that we will see actual progress and thus be reassured we will eventually move in. Someday. Hopefully before we all die; or at least, each of us is thinking, before *I* die.

IV

The Messenger: It is at that moment that the messenger soars by, a messenger bringing hope, reassurance, and freedom from fear. The messenger is feathered, flying slowly, soaring into the wind outside the glass doorway that enters onto our deck. She seems to momentarily stall in the headwind, and for that brief instant it looks as if she will land on the deck. But she sails on, tipping her wings in recognition as a fighter pilot would do to an ally, showing the full bloom of her orange-red tail.

Carlos Castaneda's Don Juan reminds us that an animal that appears at the beginning of a journey or dream sets the whole tone. In Native American lore birds – especially hawks, falcons, eagles and owls – are messengers in some form, often serving as intermediaries between humans and the Great Mystery (or Great Spirit or Creator).

All of us in the room, looking out at a horizon full of bird-wing, are on a journey – moving from active lives to retirement; from upright and spry two-leggeds to hunched over and limping; downsizing the prized possessions we've collected (and that no one wants now) to stuff that will fit into a small housing unit – a unit that will look out into at least one hawk's flyway.

V

Hawks and Us: Some say that since The Fall (the era when we humans domesticated ourselves and moved from hunter-gatherer to farmer) – since those days of yore when the animals and plants could still speak to us (and when we were still able to understand their speakings) – all the creatures of nature are just waiting for a chance, any chance, to once again talk to us so we can once more learn from them.

I don't know about all that – seems a mite unscientific to someone like me who has been poisoned by so many years of scientism propaganda. But I do know this: since we moved from the farm to town several years ago now, Sue and I have been accompanied by a hawk on nearly every walk we've taken … and our almost-daily walks are on Lawrence city sidewalks that are bordered almost every step of the way by edge-of-town apartments and/or suburban housing developments.

Our accompaniment of hawks has been a veritable menagerie: Mostly Red-tails of course; an occasional Cooper's or Sharp-Shinned (don't ask me to tell them apart); a summertime visit from a Northern Harrier, skimming the grasses on the one open field we walk along; a wee Kestrel looking down at us in disapproval. And then a surprise look-see from a Red-shouldered hawk, a bird I did not have on my life list, but one that is moving up from the south into Kansas thanks to climate change.

We see our hawks sitting elegantly upright in trees, on telephone poles, on roofs (including our Village complex). Mostly though, we see them as dots in the sky, soaring on high, using their wings as sails in the winds.

Now I honestly don't know if the hawks follow me, or am I just more observant than I once was? But at my age, it matters not one whit. I am NOT a hawk whisperer, nor do I have any special mystical, magical power. I simply watch for the hawks … and then I honor them by talking to them as if their spirit were a part of mine; which is exactly how I feel.

Perhaps it is that, by a simple act of showing respect, a soaring part of nature notices and rewards that respect with its presence. That's all I can hope for.

VI

A New Journey: It's now been several years since our meeting with our Red-tailed Hawk, and a lot has transpired. Shortly after that hawk soared by our windows, I was diagnosed with Stage IV prostate cancer and had surgery to remove a tumor on my spine … and thus a new journey began for me. We have moved into the Villages and have found it to be a magical place with a flock of good, caring folks to chat and commune with.

The hawks have remained – seen along the way on my wobbly saunterings and occasionally soaring by our new home's windows to the world.

This past Christmas we sent a hawk poster to Taylor, the granddaughter who wants it to inspire her to further heights as she plays volleyball at Northern Colorado. In exchange, her mother (our daughter, Kim) gave us a metal Peregrine falcon to mount on the driftwood we have fastened to our deck – our idea of an art project.

VII

More Hawk: Life is good. Sue and I are returning from a small get-together of Village folk, and I settle into my easy chair, turning the TV on.

Sue hisses: "Oh my god! Randy, turn around slowly, very slowly. But hurry!"

I do as instructed, and Oh my god! There is a hawk, a huge hawk, a living hawk, sitting on the driftwood at the corner of our deck where we plan to eventually mount the metal hawk. Our red tailed friend just sits there, evidently happy with her perch. She is staring out, toward the parking lot, seemingly not bothered by us or the TV.

I fumble into my pants pocket, retrieve the phone, and shaking like a cottonwood leaf, flick to camera mode. As I am clicking away, our hawk slowly, very slowly, turns its head and stares directly into the camera. She stays on her perch for what seems like a short lifetime, then slowly and elegantly moves into flight mode, hops once, and as she falls off into the twilight air, extends wings and soars out and away.

VIII

Last Words: "Ho Mitakuye Oyasin. Be well, mighty friend. Be well, and we will also try to stay well as we begin our next journey, dealing with whatever tomorrow's challenges will be."

Chapter 18 Interlude: Tone-Setting Hawks

I

Tone-Setting Hawks: Throughout my entire life, Nature has been there – much as Castaneda's Don Juan Mateus reminded us – to set the tone for my next journey. But Hawk has become a particular tone-setter here of late – and especially here lately as I take on life's final journey.

Hawk was there when we moved from country to city. Hawk was there as we struggled with our new living arrangements; there when we journeyed through Covid's pandemic, and there as we bared arms for the vaccine jabs. Hawk was there when our new living quarters were flooded thanks to crappy construction; and most importantly, there when I got the word that I had prostate cancer.

Hawk has also been there for most of my short, daily journeys, walking along sidewalks as I try to ride out the cancer and the anti-cancer drug symptoms. Simply put: Hawk has been there for my life's difficult and long journeys and been there for the short and enjoyable ones.

Given our human propensity for a helter skelter lifestyle, it can be a bit confusing trying to figure out which journey the hawk is there to set the tone for. And maybe that's the always-message: until our species learns how to stop, look and learn, listen, and respect … our stabilizing gyroscope will always be just a little bit askew.

Even the hawks, as they were joining me for my multitude of journeys, seemed to be a mite confused. They often seem to be asking as they are soaring along with me on my various journeys: Do I encourage this journey, discourage it, or just go along for the ride?

And finally, as I opt for Hospice – because I see no reason to be barely-alive-but-totally-befogged – the hawks have once again appeared to help me on this, my next and final journey.

II

Hawks After Hospice: Soon after I opt for Hospice, Sue and I are out walking together when we notice a pair of Red-tails soaring high above us. And these two seem to be circling around us as we walk.

This is the season for lust among most species, and hawks are not above being smitten. So, there they are: two hawks, up in the sky, riding the winds, trying to impress each other. Or are they trying to impress us – hawks riding the airwaves are Nature's natural emissaries for connecting us, ground to sky.

As we turn the final corner leading to our Village Co-op, we stop to watch. I can feel Sue's steadying hand on my back, a necessary stabilizer for my wobbly proprioception – necessary whenever I try to look up.

One of the pair seems to split from his task of impressing the other (or us), and he drops down to about 100 feet above ground. His circling becomes suddenly tighter, and then the wing collapses, the nosedive into a full throated, 100 mph stoop, the silver flash of bird-lightning in action.

The flash of bird-stoop hits the ground of an abandoned farm-site next to our Village Co-op. Immediately after ground contact, a quick gathering of wings and talons, a leap and one wing beat, then two and three … and he is back airborne – holding a prize of some sort in his talons.

So, what's the message here? Well, one message could be: "You're in for one hell-of-a dive, Big Fella. Be Prepared!" Or it could be something like: "Big Guy, you may be in for some big dives as you're navigating this next journey … but look for the reward at the end of those dives, and you'll be OK."

That's what I love about messages from Nature: They are so full of great mysteries.

The next day I am walking alone along another trail that takes me by Pond 1 and the geese living there. I sneak up to the fence so I can see if Goose is nesting yet. As I am doing my best sneak-along, a Red-tail takes off from somewhere down in the pond area.

And Red-tail sets some sort of tone for my next life's journey … by screaming at me in hoarse hawk tones: Kee-eeeee-ar, kee-eeeee-ar, kee-eeeee-ar. These screams are then interrupted by a series of shrill chwirk, chwirk, chwirks … then back to the kee-eeeee-arr-ing.

Hawk continues these shouted admonitions the entire time she is climbing to soaring altitude. Then, ghost-like, she becomes a dot in the sky and disappears. This whole time (several minutes) I've had my back leaned up against the fence for stability … and now I'm plumb dizzy.

Well, what's the message here? I've never had a hawk talk to me like this before. Was she just pissed off that I interrupted whatever she was doing? Or was there a different, more succinct, maybe even more sacred, message within all that screeching.

III

Last Words: Ah, to be able to talk with the animals once again.

Geese

I

Goose Talk: It is early March, about nine months into living with cancer, and I am walking in the twilight of evening. There is a chilly mist in the air; the streetlights which appear suddenly out of the mist are adorned with a spooky halo. I hear a honking from behind. One honk. Two. Then several in a row. I think it is someone I know, honking to get my attention. I turn to see, trip, and topple to the right, using my walking stick to avoid a fall.

Then, out of the mist, the honker is right there, an apparition from the heavens. Directly overhead. If I could still jump as high as I once could, or if I could jump at all, I could touch her feathers. I watch as she wings straight for the pond, circles twice, sets up for her final approach into the wind, lowers landing gear, and glides to a graceful, two-point, web-footed landing atop the waters of MegaMart's retention pond.

I walk up to the fence, carefully keeping a tree between me and the pond. She stands there, down at the pond's edge, honking non-stop. I leave so as not to disturb her. Hopefully, she will be there tomorrow, and I hope beyond hope, her honking will have attracted her mate.

Well, hope beyond hope is eventually fulfilled, and I will be visiting, watching, and learning from goose, gander, and (eventually) their brood of goslings over this coming summer ... and for several summers to come.

II

The Family: Since that early introduction to Goose, for the last four years, each of the two retention ponds on my walking route has become summer home to a pair of Canada geese, and I've done my best to become the goose whisperer for each of the pairs. I am respectful of their private lives and tiptoe to the fences at the edge of the ponds, trying not to disturb them. I speak to them softly in warm tones and tell them that I appreciate them and that I wish them well. They occasionally look my way, but for the most part, ignore me.

Sometimes, I am able to sneak into position for a hurried photo-op of the geese; but they are generally at the edge of being photogenic, just outside the limits of my cell phone's camera lens. Most results are fuzzy images of feather lumps, hanging out in green grassy stuff or floating atop blue-grey waters.

Often, one of the fuzzy feather-lumps has a visible head of bold black and white, sitting regally atop a long and elegant white neck. The other fuzzy feather-lump is usually eating or lounging in the grass with its head hidden beneath a wing.

Eventually, momma goose chooses to nest in the crotch of tree roots, on a small spit of land that projects into Pond 1. The long necked, alert one is the gander, Zeus personified, acting as sentinel for the smaller, more demure nesting one. We three are on neutral, if not buddy-buddy, terms. Usually.

Composing my story of goose helps me get through the physical strain and the tedium of walking … so I can continue to lotion my joints with my motions.

On occasion, we have surprised each other – me wobbling on my walking sticks, them waddling on webbed feet – and I am greeted with much hissing, neck coiled cobra-like into the ready-to-strike position, and an irritated angry honking.

Once, while I was scanning the far horizon for their presence, there they were, walking in the grass along the sidewalk not three feet away. All three of us were startled, and I was able to back off enough to make them comfortable. Another time, I had once again walked up on one unannounced and was afraid he would flop into the fence and hurt himself. No worries – with a jump and two wing strokes he cleared the fence and then glided onto the pond.

I imagine that my goose watching ways have bonded us, the goose pair and I, into some sort of multi-species family. For the most part it seems they agree – at least they are not attacking me as an enemy. I didn't realize how strong the bond had become though, until about two months into my walking with geese and trying to write their story.

III

Goose Blubberer: I have not seen my geese for several days now, and I'm worried that something has happened to them. I had figured it was about time for the brood to be hatched, and the hatching is a critical time for any goose family. There are plenty of obstacles to raising a brood in the city: dogs, cats, coyotes, hawks, cars, stupid people who can be a constant disturbance, and more.

But when I creep up to a viewing site at the fence around the pond, there they are, down at the pond's edge: the two adults with heads held high. Whoa. What's that sneaking through the grasses? It looks like some sort of long fuzzy thing, about six inches tall.

But wait. It's not one thing; it's several thingies, things that, with the aid of my binoculars, become individual gosling fuzzballs. There are maybe five or six or seven of them – being herded and led, front of the line and the back, by momma and poppa goose.

Then, out of nowhere, some lurking danger presents itself. One honk from either goose or gander, barely audible. All hands are in immediate scurry mode – five or six or seven little fluffballs in motion all at once, scrawny arms (wings without feathers) raised overhead, skinny legs pumping as fast as foot-webbing and waddling-gait will allow. In unison, they all speed to shore's edge and one-by-one they hop and plop into the water.

Goose has preceded them; gander brings up the rear, offering a beaked prod if necessary. Goslings – thanks to the buoyancy of their fluff – bob on ripples of water like corks on a fishing line. They take immediately to the water ... and to the regimen of staying in line and minding Mom and Pop.

It seems to be an almost unstated rule of order, goose and gander are now in charge of the flotilla that swims to the middle of the pond – evidently avoiding some danger that I am never able to see, even with my binocs.

As I watch, the parents escort the youngsters to the far-side shoreline, then out of the water onto shore – the goslings struggling up the shoreline with little scrawny-fuzzy, not-yet-wings held high overhead. Goslings become little wind-waves in the grass, and momma goose eventually settles down, raises her wings to blanket her brood, and they crawl underneath, into the warmth of goose down.

IV

Blubbering: Well, that's when the blubbering begins. Damned if I know to this day where it came from. I don't cry. No male in the Kidd family ever cries. We're too frapping tough for that. But the tears start. Tears stream. I start to sob and blubber. Uncontrollably.

Gaining a little control of myself, I look around to make sure no one is watching and dry my face on my sleeves. I head for home a few hundred yards away. I open the door ... and start the blubbering all over again. Right there in front of Sue. Dagnabbit!

V

Last Words: So, what is one to make of blubbering?

Obviously, I was flummoxed by the geese and their goslings – chemo fog is a formidable mind befuddler. Maybe I've been holding in too much of the grief that goes along with being diagnosed with cancer, terminal cancer – stoicism in the face of adversity is a well-known Kidd-family trait. Also, it could be the female hormones that they have me on, working their magic and helping me become more feminine – able to cry after all.

Or maybe – maybe it was just too overwhelming, too mind-boggling, to realize that life in nature, including life in the form of fuzzy wee goslings, will continue to go on ... with or without me.

Whatever. Whatever it is, to the end of my days I will own up to my new title of Goose Blubberer, and once again I will thank nature for providing me with insights not available in my human world.

Chapter Interlude 19: Goose Families

I

World of the Goose: As I write this I've been entertained, energized, educated, and saddened over the course of four years by those two families of geese, each one living on one of the retention ponds along my walking route. Families is the keyword here: geese are the ultimate in family making and keeping.

Canada goose nesting season in Kansas begins in early to mid-March; the birds that nest here may be one of several sub-species of Canadas that travel the Central Flyway, from the upper reaches of Arctic Canada down into Texas. The geese that stay here in Kansas to nest (instead of flying on into Canada) are called "resident Canada geese."

II

Territories are staked out and the ganders are fierce protectors – Zeus in feathers, wielding a thunderbolt of biting beak along with a wingspan they use as the forearm shiver of a football lineman ... fending off competitors who are vying for the wing of their beloved.

First, there is the dare: lowered head, stretched out and down to water level and aimed directly at the interloper. Then, if that doesn't work, the flying run across the top of the water – a thunderbolt in action, skimming the water surface. Next, if the intruding swain hasn't already flown away, the head and beak, coiled as a snake, ready to strike; and then, finally, the contact – with lots of chasing, biting, and pulling of tail feathers, and ultimately the shivered-wing beat-down. The smack down of gander!

Winner takes all. Mother goose has taken it all in from afar, calmly grazing on the greening grasses. She awaits the courting ... which also involves flamboyant displays of extended wing-span, undignified flopping of wings, and considerable running and dancing on the top of the water.

End result: 5 to 7 eggs, huge and startlingly white, laid about

1.5 days apart. With her full clutch of eggs in the nest, goose sits on them for 28 days while gander, neck extended elegantly above the grasses, acts as watchdog.

Minding Mom and Pop: Only rarely do I see any need for corporeal punishment or even raised voices. Mom and Pop are in charge of protecting their little ones. Little ones, obey ancient instincts, following the lead of parents who care.

I will watch the little ones grow into teenagers, long and lean; then into young adults with fully-feathered attire. In goose land, this all takes about two months. And then the babies, now able to fly, do just that – they fly away to parts unknown to me. To start their lifecycle all over again.

III

Last Words: Four years of watching goose cycles and I think I get it now. Families are about taking care of and then instilling actionable know-how that will help the following generations in their life's journeys … for as long as the youngsters need the caretaking and the teachings. Then, when the time is right, it's time to let them go; to let them go into their own worlds of re-generation, one generation after another.

I'm not sure that geese keep track of their young after they leave the family to go it on their own. I do know Sue and I have been blessed to be able to keep tabs on all our young'uns, and all their youngsters, and the young brood that marks the third generation to come behind us.

The tab-keeping has been well worth it. As we have been witness to the process of caring, teaching and then letting go, I can only say that it all makes me extremely proud of what our family has accomplished and become.

If I were a gander, I'd honk my head off, bragging about my kids and their kids and their kids' kids. Or I might swell my chest out, fluff my feathers and hiss like a cobra chicken.

Whatever. What I can say is that I am one very proud poppa, grandpa, and great grandpa. So proud it brings tears to my eyes.

Fog

I

Fog: Today is a foggy day. Very foggy. And I love it. Walking in the fog is refreshing – water droplets bathing and cooling skin, befogging glasses, matting down hair. I suppose it's the Irish in me; an ancient genetic code that relishes the reality and the mythology of mists, of fogs, of clouds.

Fog is, in reality, a cloud that has reached down to touch the ground. Thus, as we walk into the fog, we are metaphorically "walking on clouds." And those clouds we see in the sky are the ultimate "shape shifters" – giving our minds something new to imagine every step we take along the way.

Walking in the fog is, for me, a joy. Perhaps it's the mystery of what lies around the fog-hidden corner. Perhaps it is that you see more critters along the way – big eyes peering out from their hiding place behind the shroud of fog. At least it *seems* as if you see more critters.

Perhaps it's the quieting effect of the fog, as it wraps around all sense organs and blankets them from the hum and drum of civilization. Perhaps it's the memory of walking in the fogs of San Francisco when we lived there many years ago – thick night-time fog rolling in from the sea, always to the accompaniment of throaty foghorns sounding their warnings across the Bay. The sound of many foghorns, muted in the clouds of fog, is hauntingly mesmerizing.

And so, there is a certain beauty surrounding fog. And fog's close cousin, *mist*, has a similar, if slightly more muted, beauty and mystery about it.

II

Mist: Instead of fog, I could just as easily be walking in and enjoying mist – they are the same phenomenon, fog just a denser variety of mist. So, you have almost exactly the same feeling, walking in mist or in fog, but when it comes to mystery and mystical tales, me thinks mist has a wee bit of an advantage over fog.

Perhaps it's just that *mist* has a more lyrical ring to it than does *fog*. (Try saying them both out loud, and you'll hear what I mean.) And perhaps it's this resonance of sound-to-lyrics that the Irish poets so often rely upon to create a poem both melancholic and optimistic.

To be sure, both fog and mist have the same literal meaning: water in the form of droplets floating or falling in the atmosphere at or near the surface of the earth and approaching the form of rain. For those of scientific mind, mist is less-thick fog. *Fog* is the name given to resulting visibility less than one kilometer (1,093.6 yards or 0.621371 miles); on a *misty* morn, you can still see things at least 1000 meters (one kilometer) down the trail.

III

Haze, Smoke, and Smog are additional terms that, when spoken aloud, sound much harsher than fog, or mist, or cloud. It could be that they sound harsher ... because they are harsher.

Haze is composed of small dry particles in the air that, by themselves, are invisible ... until together they become a dense enough congregation to make the sky appear as if it is shrouded in a thin veil of milky gauze, glittering in the sunlight. *Smoke* is, of course, created when something is burned ... and the ashes from the burning reach into the skies. *Smog* is a term created in the early 1900's to describe the combination of smoke and fog – a sooty combination that had, by then, become a common phenomenon around areas populated heavily by humans.

And so be it for the realities behind the additives to our skies; for me the real interest lies in the stories – the symbology, mythologies and mysteries – we have built around them.

IV

Watery Skies: I suppose we should expect any alteration to our skies to carry within it some mysterious symbology along with its resultant mythological story. Humans have always looked to the skies for spiritual guidance, and a guide that can seemingly shape-shift at will is certainly worthy of being the creator of stories.

Childhood is a time to lie on your back, look up into the clouds, and make up your own stories as to what wild creatures you are seeing and what they are doing. Or at least it should be your time for that. The stories you can tell your young mind are constantly changing as the clouds move across the horizon, as they shift from one shape to another.

Here in Kansas even the adults watch the clouds as they are constantly shifting – hoping that the next winds don't bring in the rotating wall cloud buried in ominous green skies – skies punctuated by lightning bolts thrown by Zeus or, in another story, that have come from the beak of the Thunderbird. Kansans know that this kind of sky can quickly turn into the full-blown tornado that transports Dorothy and Toto into another world.

It's no surprise, then, that clouds have many metaphorical meanings – for novelists, playwrights, and songwriters (and memoirists). For these, as well as for poets and philosophers, watery skies (clouds and fog and mist) may be the most useful metaphors of all time.

You can make a cloud or mist or fog be a character in your story. Or any of them can stand for bad things (a love affair gone bad, for one example, or as a philosophy with bad consequences). Or they can represent something hidden … or something that needs to hide. And they can be used to stand in for any of the many incarnations of a soul.

Or in modern times, the cloud may be where reams of data are stored – a storage that involves huge human-built warehouse areas and massive computer servers that are powered and cooled by mechanically-induced energetics.

V

Last Words: And so, me thinks that clouds and mists and fog offer metaphors too vast to wrap our heads around, too elusive to ever catch up to, too squiggly to ensnare in any web we might cast, were we ever able to run them down.

I turn to Joni Mitchel's "Both Sides Now" to help me understand clouds and fog and mist a bit better. To recognize that maybe the best we can do is to realize that it is, after all, life's illusions we really recall. Reality is, and will always be, shrouded within the clouds and fogs and mists Nature creates for us.

"I really don't know life at all." Line from "Both Sides Now" — by Joni Mitchel.

Chapter 20 Interlude: Chemo Smog

I

Chemo Fog: There is one type of fog that does not wear a happy face: chemofog (or chemobrain). And wouldn't you know it would also (like all things medical) have an acronym: CRCI (chemotherapy-related cognitive impairment) or CICI (chemotherapy-induced cognitive impairment).

Chemofog is a condition that infests a heavy majority of all patients undergoing chemotherapy. Like – depending somewhat on the drug being used – upwards of 75% of all cancer patients … but almost all chemo drugs have negative cognitive effects on a majority of patients. Even worse, the foggy brain may last for months or even years after treatment ends. (Studies show that chemofog lingers for more than a few months in approximately 35% of all patients.)

II

Me the Befogged: I've had two separate rounds of chemo, and my brain fog was mild during the first round; then it lasted for several months after ending that round. (Yeah, I know, I know: how does someone already with foggy mind determine it was the chemo that caused an even foggier brain? Stay with me here.)

It took several months after that first round for me to get most of my thinking abilities back. And to be honest, I didn't fully realize how much cognitive ability I had lost until I was off chemo for several months … and the old mental-me began to slowwwwly return. Turns out chemofog comes in on pussytoes and then silently haunches down, ready to pounce when least expected.

My second round of chemo just plain-and-simple knocked me out. I couldn't think, couldn't sleep, couldn't walk without taking time to focus on "one foot after another." I had a hard time remembering Sue's name. I'm a couple of months post chemo now, and I still find myself sitting and staring into a foggy horizon – wondering where I am, who I am, and why I am.

III

Symptoms: Cancer patients can tell you, often in vivid detail, the cognitive changes they have suffered as they were on chemo: the often-debilitating problems with memory, thinking and concentration. Common symptoms include: difficulty concentrating and decreased attention span, disorganized thinking, an inability to focus, difficulty making decisions, confusion, word recall difficulties, lack of mental clarity, requiring more time to finish routine tasks, difficulty retaining new information, and difficulty with visual or verbal memory.

Veterinarians have a term for this: "ADR" as in "That dog's an ADR (Ain't Doin' Right)... with the usual addition of "and I have no idea why he ain't doin right nor what we should do about it."

Oncologists can only shrug when asked what chemo fog really is ... or how to cure it. And while they make it a point to give much lip service to Quality of Life (QoL) concerns, they continue to use drugs that literally destroy QoL ... all in the name of adding on a few extra months of life.

IV

Chemofog Is: There have just recently (finally!) been some studies trying to ferret out the causes of chemofog and perhaps come up with a mechanism to improve quality of life.

Studies have shown that chemotherapies muddle up our ability to think by churning our brain cells. Apparently all of our brain cells – including the poetically-named oligodendrocytes, astrocytes, microglia, and neurons – are affected.

The muddling is brought on by a variety of biochemical reactions which may act in several different ways, including: 1) reducing blood flow to the brain which negatively affects brain glucose metabolism and cognition; 2) diminishing the development of new nerve cells – ultimately resulting in fewer individual nerve cells and an overall depletion of white matter; and 3) creating an imbalance or dysregulation of several cellular biochemicals – with resulting toxic effects to individual cells and to the body's immunological system in general.

Bottom line: chemo-drugs are toxic to inner parts of nerve cells. The toxicity affects the growth and regeneration of nerve cells and/or causes cellular damage and death. Healthy nerve cells are turned into a milky mush of cell debris and body fluids – mush and debris which not only clouds thinking; but also mush that must be removed before we can clear up our thinking.

So, Nature's clouds and mists and fogs basically coddle and caress us, body, mind and soul. Contrariwise, using chemotherapies is like pouring a thick cloud of fog into the cranium and then stirring chunks of dead cellular stuff into the cloud – kinda like starting a fire on a foggy day and watching as the ashes and fog mix together to create a toxic smog.

Perhaps we should be calling it chemosmog instead of chemofog. Then we could say we were smogged instead of fogged – which I think has a more accurate ring to how it really feels.

V

Managing Chemofog: OK, so we're getting closer to understanding the biochemical reasons for the chemofog, and from this perhaps we'll be able to devise a silver bullet to cure it. In the meantime a few things have been recognized as being helpful: exercise, nutrition, and maintaining an actively working brain.

Wait. What? You mean that exercise – the very activity that is made much more difficult by the chemotherapies that cause weight gain, lymphedema, severe fatigue, and swelling and pain of joints (and in my case swelling of scrotum) – could be a cure for chemofog … if you could use it. What a concept. Maybe motion is lotion after all.

And you say that proper nutrition also helps prevent chemofog … because chemo drugs, in addition to impacting the central nervous system, disrupt the healthy gut-brain axis. The resulting microbiota imbalance can cause visceral discomfort, intestinal permeability, and changes to the body's immunological systems.

And so, while we're spending all our time looking for the silver bullet cancer cure, perhaps we should also be helping patients achieve a healthy microflora.

And, while cognitive therapies have had variable results for cancer patients, brainy scientists say it never hurts to encourage patients to engage in activities that make their brains work ... even though those types of activities have become nigh-on impossible due to the chemofog.

VI

Last Words: Well, I'll be damned. Once again, it looks as if we've had our thinking besmogged by institutions that were originally created to serve mankind ... but have, over time, become institutions we are obliged to serve.

Mullein

I

Introduction: I'm looking back to several decades ago. We have recently moved our family from San Francisco onto a small acreage in Kansas, and I am in graduate school, trying to decipher the foreign language of veterinary clinical pathology.

We are hoping that the move to the country will give our daughters a better feel for the outdoors and nature ... but are discovering that milking goats, "harvesting" (aka butchering) chickens and rabbits, and doing daily farm chores is **not** what they had in mind for their high school years.

It is a dark and blustery early-autumn Kansas day – spitting snow/rain/sleet/hail. I am staring out the window facing south, absentmindedly watching a small herd of deer browsing out there. They seem to be intent on munching on one particular plant, one that is easy to see as it sticks up, head-high, above the grasses. I mark one of the plants for later investigation and go back to my studies.

It takes some serious time in the veterinary library to ID the plant the deer are so interested in, but I eventually find it in one of those books of Kansas noxious weeds: it is mullein, *Verbascum Thapsus*. According to the book, if you find it in your fields, mullein is not especially difficult to get rid of. I wonder what the deer see in a noxious weed ... so I continue to investigate.

My investigations eventually lead me to the study of herbology and to many years of using herbal medicines for my animal patients.

II

Mullein: Mullein is one of those troublesome Eurasian plant imports, brought over by trouble-making European pilgrims – perhaps as seedy stowaways hidden in ships' provisions or in a trouble-maker's pants cuffs. An adult mullein produces thousands of seeds, each the size of a salt granule, and each seed easily scattered by the winds.

Once you've been properly introduced, mullein is an easy plant to ID: 1) it is a biennial plant with first year growth as a low-lying rosette of broad, lance-shaped leaves, and 2) the second year's growth sends it upwards of six feet or more. The second year's growth sprouts a stout stalk capped off with a cob-like spear that is surrounded by small yellow flowers.

III

Medicinal Mullein: Once our backyard deer had introduced me to mullein, I had a bad case of "The Wonders." I wondered why the deer were so hungry for it during those early, cold days of fall.

Easy answer: Mullein has a long history of being used as a mild sedative and tonic for lung and bronchial problems, including: colds, hay fever, asthma, spasmodic coughing, sore throat, acute respiratory infection, and hoarseness, whooping cough and other bronchial symptoms.

OK, so that's why *we humans* use mullein, especially during the fall season when lung and bronchial problems are common. But what about the deer? How have they learned about the medicinal qualities of mullein? And more importantly, without libraries full of books-for-deer, how have they been able to pass their knowledge on to the following generations?

My guess is that it was the deer who somehow figured out the medicinal qualities of mullein … and then we learned from them, by watching them. But the question remains: how did the deer "somehow figure out" the medicinal qualities of mullein? Trial and error? Seems like that would take forever, but it's possible.

What about a larger Nature Spirit, possibly working at a genetic level to help assure the survival of the species? And perhaps this Spirit works subtly by making the mullein taste like deer candy in the fall, and only during the fall. Then, as the deer munch away on their candy, they bump into the seed heads, knock seeds asunder, and those seeds get scattered by the winds … and everyone lives happily ever after.

And so, these are the thoughts and questions I took with me into my beginnings of becoming an herbalist … after watching the deer lead the way.

IV

More Mullein Meds: The study of herbs (many of which are common "weeds") can prod the student to walk many pathways that have, for centuries now (and for most of us), been over-grown by the weeds of disregard, disrespect, and disuse. These are, of course, the same pathways that have been long-trodden by scores of others: the herbalists that have come before us.

Herbal studies can also open the gateways that allow for a neuronal trailblazing of sorts – new thinking emanating from the roots, stems, leaves and flowers of the plants. New ways of seeing the world via the nature of wisdom that is inherent with-in the plants.

Look further into mullein, for example, and you will find a wealth of uses, both traditional and relatively new. Mullein tea made from the leaves has not only been used as a lung and bron-chial herb; it has also been used to treat gastrointestinal cramps and urinary conditions including bed wetting.

A tea made from mullein flowers has been used to induce sleep or to reduce pain or headache, and the flowers in an oil in-fusion can be used to treat ear infections. Mullein flower oil was one of my favorite remedies for treating chronic ear infections in dogs.[15]

Mullein has been put to use in other, rather odd-ball ways. For example, early farmers used a smudging smoke from the dried leaves as a barn "cleansing" agent – preparing the barn and its inhabitants for the winter. Leaves have been used as a

---

15 I used the entire flower "cob" (including flowers), cut into smaller pieces – picking individual flowers is too much effort for lazy old me. Place flowers and cob pieces into a small jar; cover with oil and let sit for a week or so. If you want to, you can add some St John's wort and/or a garlic clove for a bit more potency. Strain. Use a dropper or so of the oil in affected ears.

I found this remedy very effective in my veterinary practice – and I understand that it appears to be equally effective for human children with earaches. AND, rather than being irritating (as are many remedies), mullein oil actually seems to have a soothing effect.

poultice to remove warts and treat other skin conditions.

One of the out-of-the-past locally-common names for mullein was "Quaker's Rouge." Supposedly there was a time when Quaker ladies were forbidden to use facial makeup. But, being ever-resourceful, they had discovered that a quick rub with the leaves of mullein would provide a nice red flush to the cheeks.

And finally (my favorite, and another example of using the plant on cheeks): mullein leaves (fluffy soft and wide enough to be useful) are, to this day, known hereabouts as *"Cowboy Toilet Paper."*

Now a lot of these uses might appear a mite hokey in today's world of science, but mullein leaves and flowers were officially listed in the National Formulary from 1916-36, classifications as a demulcent – the leaves were also classified as emollient and flowers as pectoral. Proving once again that there's nothing like tagging something with a Latin name to give it sachet and credibility.

V

Mullein's Ancient History: With a list of uses like that above, you might expect that mullein has a long history of being considered a very useful plant … and you'd be right. In medieval times mullein was known as the "Herb of Love" or the "Herbe of Protection", and it is likely the "moly" that Mercury gave Ulysses to use as a charm against Circe's enchantments.

In 7th Century Europe mullein was named "herbe de St. Fiacre", after the Irish saint who became the patron saint of all gardeners: Saint Fiacre of Breuil (c. AD 600 - 670). (If you are at all interested in gardening or medicinal plants, the tale of St. Fiacre is a story about a dude you absolutely must get to know.) And then, going up a level from a mere priest and hermit-gardener, mullein's other common names include: Aaron's rod; and Jacob's and St. Peter's staff – all of which introduce follow-up stories worth pursuing.[16]

---

16 Saint Fiacre is the patron of growers of vegetables and medicinal plants, and gardeners in general. His reputed aversion to women is believed to be the reason that he is also considered the patron of victims of venereal disease. He is further the patron of victims of hemorrhoids and fistulas, taxi cab drivers, box makers, florists, hosiers, pewterers, tilemakers, and those suffering from infertility. Finally, he is commonly invoked to heal persons suffering from various infirmities, premised on his reputed

VI

Last Words: And so, watching deer munch on mullein has led me down many a pathway. I figured that if the deer and mullein could teach me something about medicine, I should pay attention.

Chapter 21 Interlude: Mullein My Sentinel

I

Weed Doctor: In addition to mullein, I used a lot of local "weeds" in my holistic veterinary practice, including: dandelion, plantain, echinacea, hawthorn berries, licorice root, and more. And so, I wear the title of "weed doctor" with pride.

Along the way, I've met a lot of very kindly mentors who have helped me on my learning journeys – mentors that have included plants, animals (wild and tame), and herbalists. As mentor-teachers, I've found that all of these use a soft and easy approach to teaching, making it extremely easy for the learner to learn.

In addition to my gurus being soft and easy, I've mostly thought of the herbs as nice, mild "medicines" that, rather than forcing themselves into pathways of the body's healing mechanisms, they simply helped my patient's inner body heal itself.

In addition, looking into the histories of the plants as healers has given me many hours of enjoying the stories that the saints, sinners, and really smart people have to tell.

II

Plants As Sentinels: Finally, there's one final "use" of mullein that comes out of Native American lore. Several tribes believe that mullein is a sentinel plant (some tribes include poison ivy as a sentinel) – a plant that pokes its head up and looks around to see if it's safe for other plants to follow. Sentinels are given respect and allowed to grow to show other plants where they

---

skill with medicinal plants. (from Wikipedia)

too might be welcomed.[17]

In today's world mullein is easy to find in an area where recent construction has occurred. For example, the city recently cut a path through a small cedar grove – first dozing the trail, then laying down a layer of pea-gravel. It is one of my favorite trails, and this is the first spring after the dozing…and huge, fuzzy leaves of first-year mullein plants can be seen everywhere along the trail.

My take on this is that dozing the path was, for the land, akin to one of us scraping our knees in a fall. Whereas we might put a bandage on our scrape, Nature might instead provide a soft, fluffy leaf-bearing plant for protection while She looks around to see if it's safe for other plants to grow in the area.

And I remember that, in my case, it was the deer – munching on our area's mullein plant – that had created a sentinel for me – so that I then had the confidence to learn and practice herbal medicine (and eventually other alternative medicines including homeopathy, chiropractic, and acupuncture) for my animal patients.

III

Last Words: Thank you, my Sentinels. Thank you for being there when I needed you.

---

17 Etymologists think sentinel stems from the Old Italian words sentina, meaning "vigilance," and sentire, "to hear or perceive." It's a close cousin of sentry, which means the same thing. You can use sentinel as a noun or a verb. A kid in a snowball war might be the sentinel, patrolling the entrance to the fort. (Vocabulary.com)

Murmurations

I

Introduction: We often look to the sky for inspiration: the artistic hues of sunrise and sunset; clouds that can tell entire stories while we lie on our backs and let our imaginations soar; the coming of weather on the horizon – good omen skies or ones more foreboding, aflame with lightning and rumbling with thunder. But there is nothing more inspiring of awe and astonishment than a murmuration of starlings.

II

A Murmuration of Starlings: A symphony of movement – from several hundred to as many as several million black birds representing gazillions of moving parts, all aswirl. Huge flocks of birds forming dense spheres, ellipses, columns, and vibrating lines, and then changing shape within moments. Black dots against the pale light of morning or evening sky – yin/yang in motion. Tornadoes of birds, their vortex undulating from side to side, up to down. A breath of wings and feathers, expanding, contracting, throbbing as the pulse of a sky full of heart.

A mass of birds with a purpose – or many purposes. A flock moving to roost, moving to confuse predators, moving to stay warm, to socialize, to find food, to tell their buddies where to find food – moving to delight the observer, to delight themselves.

Murmurations are typically seen in the evenings, during the winter months, from October to March, with a peak in numbers usually occurring in December and January. Murmurations are a phenomenon of European starling flocks; and those European birds that were introduced to the U.S. have gradually taken up the habit. A typical murmuration in this country is composed mostly of starlings – with a scattering of other black birds, including red wing black birds, grackles, and crows.

III

How They Do It: Starlings in a murmuration, according to scientists who study such things, have a sense of balance that relies on spatial distances, one bird to another ... or oftentimes to a group of seven or so birds.

Starlings seek to match the direction and speed of the seven or so neighboring birds. (Starlings are able to react in less than 100 milliseconds, and they can move at a speed of around 20 MPH, which is about the speed an average NFL wide receiver runs his routes.) Each matching movement then causes a number of downline reactions which ultimately creates the murmuration's swirl, throb, and flow.

Remember: There is a purpose to all this movement (or several purposes all intertwined) ... and these purposes are carried out in split seconds, micro seconds.

IV

The Mystery: We know a lot about the mechanics of motion and proprioception, but even though the nerves are there as a physical entity we can see and touch, exactly *how* our nervous system works in all of its intricate interactions is still quite a bit of a mystery.

Exactly how and what acts as the starling's nervous system and its control panel – the thing that produces murmurations – is likewise still a mystery.

I like to think that the mystery behind murmurations is simple energetics – energies between individual birds that feed, bird-to-bird, into a coordinated wave of motion that is an organism in itself, an organism without skin or spine. Thus the starlings' composite of nervous systems, acting as a flock-of-nerves, becomes the interacting murmuration.

In the human animal, this innate energetic has been called many things, but to me it looks a whole lot like *chi*, the life force of Chinese medicine.

V

Me the Murmurator: Ah, but that I could make my body parts move in such manner. I try to imagine how it might feel, if I were the murmurator, moving. The human body is, after all, composed of some 270 bones, 360 joints, and a total cell count of somewhere between 15 to 35 trillion cells – numbers rivaling those of all the moving parts of a murmuration.

But the beauty, majesty, and mystery of movement is not in the numbers; it is in the coordination of parts of the whole.

There is a beauty of movement within the athletic human body, a certain grace and flow of all body parts working in sync. Look closely at the athlete and you will see beauty in the structure of the body, much like that beauty that reveals itself to the work of the sculptor's chisel – beauty appearing, as if by magic, from within the stone. Look closely at the flow of the athletic body in action and you may be able to visualize both the grace of the body and the energetics of the spirit within that body.

VI

Last Words: Murmurations hereabouts are not nearly as huge as those seen in Europe. Still, it's pretty cool watching dozens (or perhaps a few hundred) birds gyrate in unison – filling a corner of our Kansas horizon with the beauty of their movements. (The internet has some great videos of the huge European starling murmurations.)

Anyway, when I'm out walking, I'm not out looking for any one thing in particular. My true interest is in what I can see along the way, what parts of Nature will be there for me to see, hear, smell, feel, taste ... and then to tell a story about.

Maybe today I'll see a pair of starlings breeding on the roof of one of the houses I'm walking by, or a flock of grackles arguing over the food morsel one of them has found, or a crow chasing a hawk, or a group of starlings chasing a crow, or a red wing blackbird chattering at me to let me know this is his patch of cattails.

Chapter 22 Interlude

I

The Mechanics of "Human Murmuration:" The human body in motion balances itself by relying on a number of factors, all related to proprioception.

Proprioception: the perception or awareness of the position, movement, and action of the body. It encompasses a complex of sensations, including perception of joint position and movement, muscle force, and effort. These sensations arise from signals of sensory receptors in the muscle, skin, and joints, and from central signals related to motor output. Moving at speeds of 80 to 120 meters per second, our nerves that transmit touch and proprioception are the fastest in the body.

Proprioception enables us to judge limb movements and positions, force, heaviness, and stiffness. It combines with other senses to help us locate external objects relative to the body. Proprioception could be thought of as the command center in charge of our body's physical movements ... or as the gyroscope that, when spinning, keeps us upright and on course.

The purpose of proprioception is to keep the spine and joints of the extremities aligned in such fashion that makes it easy for muscles to lever, bones around joints, to create movement ... and to keep the moving human from falling flat on his face. Proprioception, in effect, is the stimulus that tells the body's parts how to coordinate, how to stay in sync with the others – much as a murmuration of birds relies on coordination of direction that determines the space between birds.

The human motivator, the driver of all that's involved in movement and proprioception, is an intricate system of nerves and nerve endings that extend from the tips of our toes and fingers to the control panel for it all: the brain. It's the brain's job to send the proper inputs to the muscles that will (hopefully) keep us upright and balanced, able to walk or run along so we can fulfill our purpose.

In addition, there is a complex web of nerves that covers all areas of the body – a web that catches all incoming sensory stimuli from the environment around us: heat and cold from sun or snow, stings from bees or other beasties, itches from stinging nettles to pollen grains, pain from biting animals or hail stones, and more.

These sensory inputs are then translated into an action response that tells our muscles and tendons how we should respond to those environmental inputs. If all is working right, the ideal response is to avoid pain and enhance pleasure.

In an anatomy lab we can tease out the nerves involved in proprioception, sensory inputs, and activation of muscle response, and we can study them under a microscope.

We can zap nerves with electrical stimuli and see which muscles the nerves activate. We can also measure how fast the electrical impulses of various nerve types travel from skin to brain and then to muscle. We have machines that can do all this for us.

II

Murmuration of Me: So, when I walk, as a nervous system that drives levers, and as a nervous system that reacts to external stimuli and internal chi, I become a *Murmuration-of-Me* that is braced by its skeleton and confined to its own skin. What if, in the end, it is these constrictions on movement – skin and bone -- that can make me look more than a little clumsy compared to the real murmuration? Danged skin and bones keep getting in the way.

I might argue that when all my body parts (or yours) are functioning in coordinated manner, we can look almost as graceful and beautifully arty as a murmuration. I find comfort from the comparison. Well, maybe not my body parts, but certainly those of a lithe gymnast or a ballerina – either of them able to twist in the air much like a murmuration.

II

Last Words: My surgeon told me after the surgery that it would be at least six months to a year before I regained my proprioception … if ever. The "if ever" has never come. I still wobble when I walk, my muscle memory has amnesia, and in airplane terminology, my visual gyroscope has gone kaput – that is, I need to have a firm visual on the horizon or I list dangerously to one side or the other.

And so, the dream of me being a murmuration in human form is way beyond being a mite far-fetched. But the real reason I walk has nothing to do with me looking like a murmuration; I walk because motion is lotion – not just to my joints, but also to every part of me, from tip of toes to the top of my balding pate.

Birding

I

Introduction: Perhaps the easiest way – and to my way of thinking, the most captivating and thus most enjoyable way – to get into Nature is bird watching (or, as the pros refer to it: "birding"). No matter where you live (unless it's on an ice glacier at the North or South Pole) there will be birds all around you.

And no matter where you live there will be a battalion of birders (mostly, according to stereotype, a battalion of little old ladies) nearby to help you learn how to become a master birder ... should you ever want that designation. According to a U.S. Fish and Wildlife Service report issued in 2021, about 45 million Americans are birders – 39 million were "around the home-birders" and 16 million were more active "away from home-birders" who traveled at least a mile to see birds.

Furthermore, resources to help you with your birding adventures abound: there's an Audubon club in almost every nook and cranny of America, and there are several magazines and apps devoted to the various how-tos of birding. Next time you see a little old lady (or little old guy like me) walking aimlessly about with binoculars in hand, you can ask them for help.

II

Best Beginner Bird: Some birds are easy to like; others not so much. Robins fall into the easy-to-like category, so it's always good to see their return as our "harbingers of springtime." Robins are also the ideal learner-birds, a perfect place to start for the beginning birder.

First off, robins are easy to identify. From robin red breast to robin egg blue, the main colors of robin are a part of our everyday lexicon.

But it's not just the colors-of-robin that make them stand out; it's also their ability to hold our attention while they patrol our lawns, hopping about and running from one wormhole to another, using the head-cock-method for locating a tasty morsel of worm. Finding her prey, spearing it with flash of beak, then tugging, tugging, tugging until she either falls over backward … or she has a squirmy, mud-filled worm in a beak-grip where she can flip it into her mouth and gulp it down with a satisfied belch.

We're drawn to robin-watching because they don't slink around and try to hide from our view – they boldly go where no other bird would dare go: strutting, hopping, and sprinting across our well-manicured suburban and downtown lawned areas, gulping worms, bugs and berries by the gullet-full.

They may even build their homesteading nests on our windowsills, in the landscaping trees of our backyards, or under the eaves of our porch. And robin nests are uniquely robin-made: sturdy of construction, with a mud and grass base and fortified with a surrounding wall of sticks.

III

Birding 101: Using Robin as our model, birding is very simple:

- Step One: Put on your hiking boots and seasonal outside gear and step outside.
- Step Two: Right foot in front of left, left in front of right, continue until you've spotted some birds. Stop to watch them.
- Step Three: Look. How big is the bird you're watching? As birds go, a robin is about mid-sized. For now you can refer to all smaller birds as LGB's (Little Grey Birds); that's what we experts call them. Much bigger birds are what you don't want to see screaming down at you as you're rubbing your sleepy eyes after a nap in the pasture.
- Step Four: Notice the birds' colors. A robin's red breast is a dead giveaway here. If you are eagle eyed, you might notice the white ring around the robin's eyes, the yellow beak, the white breast patch, and you may even spot the white feathers on the outside of their tails as they fly away.

- Step Five: Listen. Many birds, including the robin, can be identified by listening to their song.
- Step Six: Enjoy the antics of the bird. Robins are especially antic-proud, acting out their day job and playtimes in full view of we city folk. Other birds are water bound, or inhabitants of the thickets and woodlands, or so shy they're hard to spot. For now, enjoy the easy-to-watch robins; but you'll be able to find the hiding birds as you develop your bird watching skills.

OK, for all intents and purposes you can tell all your friends that you are now an advanced-beginner birder.

IV

American Robins: Robins are known as the *harbingers of spring*. Flocks of little red breasts hopping across our lawns and flitting from tree to tree (or from one eave of our house to another), picking out the best nesting site. Even though many of them have been around all winter, the arrival of migratory flocks with their splash of colors and springtime flutterings let us know that springtime is here … and that Kansas tornadoes are just around the corner.

Our robin, in many ways, has tied us to much of our original *heritage and frontier spirit.* Early settlers from England named our robin after the bird that has recently become the national bird of Britain, the European robin, *Erithacus rubecula.* (The European robin, a flashy-looking little red-breasted bird that looks much like our robin, was originally classified as a thrush, but the European bird is now considered a flycatcher.)

Comparing the two birds, our robin is a bit bigger, but by all accounts our American Robin and the European Robin, in addition to their red breasts, have other, similar characteristics. They are both tough-ass dudes (and dudettes) who, at the drop of a chirped challenge, will fight to the finish, no matter who is the challenger. (It's said that fully 10% of European Robin mortality is from fights within families – which sounds to me more like Irish families than British ones, but that may be because I'm Irish.)

On the other hand, both the American and European robins are people-friendly, with the European model being known for its ability to be trained to come to the human hand for food. American Robins are **industrious**—serious about their day job of putting food on the table, dedicated to raising a family (often producing 4 or 5 nests in one year, with each nest containing 2 to 5 eggs), and aggressively defending their household against all comers.

Ya gotta love the American Robin's Latin name. Or at least I do. How can you not love *Turdus Migratorius*—it simply rolls off your tongue … like guano off a cliffside. Turns out the name is not as easy to pigeonhole as you might think. The genus name Turdus is actually Latin for thrush. True thrushes are medium-sized mostly insectivorous or omnivorous birds in the genus *Turdus* of the wider thrush family, *Turdidae*.

Migratorius, of course, means they are a bird species that migrates, or they once did; with climate change warming up our winters, many of today's Kansas robins stick around through the winter.

What a *song* they sing! Whistled from the treetops, a rising and falling refrain, a steady rhythm of: "Cheerily, cheer up, cheer up, cheerily, cheer up!" – repeated time and time again. Often, it's the first birdsong of the morning and the last one you hear before dark.

Robins are *tasty*. OK, this one you probably will never verify. That's because our (gluttonous and greedy) forefathers who settled this country once trapped and ate them by the thousands, almost to extinction. They were easy prey: it was once common to see dozens of robins that had migrated to the south for the winter roosting in a single tree. That made it easy hunting to toss (or shotgun) a net over roosting robins. Evidently robin red breast, when fixed in a meat pie, was once a popular and tasty dinner.

Robins helped us *rethink our biblical role as stewards of the environment and the critters therein.* While passenger pigeons are our real model for how to overharvest animals into extinction, robin (and other songbird) meat had also become so popular (and so easy to come by) that forward-thinking folks decided we ought to do something to save the robins before we'd eaten them into oblivion.

Thus, the Migratory Bird Treaty Act of 1918, was enacted to protect more than 800 species of songbirds and migratory birds from overharvest (for meat and/or feathers). Under the Act it is illegal to "pursue, hunt, take, capture, kill, or sell" a migratory bird or any of its parts, including nests, eggs, and feathers. The Act has been modified over the years, and its overall goal is to offer birds some protection from humans.

V

Robin Folklore: Robin and her red breast pop up in many tales of yore. For example, folklore stories place the robin at the manger where she either protected baby Jesus from a fire grown too big, or she fanned a warming fire that was about to die. Or the red is the lingering blood from a painful thorn she plucked from the crown on the head of Jesus on the cross ... or it's the result of robin's fluttering ministrations to the bleeding sword wounds Jesus endured. Red, the color of fire and blood.

VI

Last Words: Robins are a good starting place for beginning birders. But once they've captured your eye, you'll learn that most birds have the unique ability to both entertain and, at the same time, to help reconnect us to Nature.

Chapter 23 Interlude:
How Do She Do That

I

S cientist Sees Robin and wants to know how a bird with a brain the size of a nut finds the worm. Scientist watches Robin hopping along on a lawn. Robin stops, cocks her head both ways, listens or stares for a few seconds, then dives her beak into the ground ... pulls back, sometimes falling over backwards with the effort, as if on stage, acting in a comedic routine. But invariably, there it is, comedy or not: a fat, juicy earthworm.

Scientist decides to perform a study asking whether the robin sees, hears, smells, or feels the worm ... discovers that Robin does not like to be studied by a human with the brain the size of a coconut.

Several scientific studies find that robins will eat almost anything, regardless how fetid its smell ... so using the sense of smell to find the worm is ruled out. A robin could feel the worm underfoot ... but that's not likely, at least to the coconut-brained ones.

Several studies, using extremely sensitive sound recorders, capture the sounds of earthworms crawling through the soil and note that robins could locate the worms by listening to worm-noise. Other studies, using fake worms and worm segments that are not visible to the human eye, find that Robin can see them and thus find her meal by seeing it.

So, take your pick: either the robin sees her worm or hears it ... or both.

II

ESP: Further, while the possibility of using ESP to find the worms is mentioned by at least one scientist, it is more of a joke than as something to take seriously. But here's the thing about ESP or any other supposed airy-fairy extrasensory ability: so long as we continue to make fun of it and poo-poo its possibilities (and all the ways of perception other than those we humans have and that we can measure), we will never be able to realize its potentials.

I remind the coconut heads that being sight-dominant has diminished many of our primary senses that other animals use to decipher their day. As but one example of many, a dog's sense of smell is up to 100,000 times more powerful than a human's. And dogs hear noises at a much higher frequency (up to 45,000 Hertz), than us humans (we struggle to hear anything above about 23,000 Hertz).

Many species (some with brains even smaller than nuts) use pheromones as their primary way to orient to their environment.

Ants and snakes, as examples, lay down pheromone trails for their colony or hibernaculum mates to follow – creating trails to food, sex, and/or safety.

And how about migratory animals – birds and butterflies, for example? Scientists are still trying to unravel the mystery of a mechanism of travel that doesn't involve a GPS or Omni system. Is migration totally reliant on the magnetic forces of the earth or the position of sun and stars, or something even more airy-fairy? Perhaps only the man in the moon knows.

III

Last Words: And so it goes for Nature and her inscrutable ways – that are … well, inscrutable.

I think of my cancer and how Science's very first response was to attack it (as they attack all cancers) with a veritable armamentarium of poisons and hormone killers – all relying on the metaphors of war.

And I wonder, what if? What if Science had, at the onset of trying to "cure" cancer, what if they had used Nature's ability to use (perhaps non-measurable) inscrutable ways to achieve their goals? If their metaphors early-on had been changed from war to Nature, would we be using entirely different ways of treating cancer today? Maybe a robin could tell us … if we'd only listen.

Cattails, *Typha spp.*

I

Rebel High Schoolers: There's a side-story for why I like taking a particular route on my walk. It was one of the first ones I walked after my cancer surgery, a flat route with a ditch filled with cattails located at about the midway point of the walk.

Early on, Sue often accompanied me on my walks (in case I took a fall and couldn't get up), and so the two of us would occasionally stop and watch the sway of the cattails in the ditch. Or, we'd cross the road to see if there were any geese or red winged blackbirds or muskrats working the cattail-lined retention-pond on the other side of the road – the Thin Place that I refer to as my Pond Two.

The ditch is the drain for my Pond Two, feeding into the sewer system that eventually empties into the Kaw River several miles north. The ditch and the pond offer a wonderful meditative respite from my walking … and a chance to catch my breath and to get my legs back under me.

But the real reason I have a personal affinity for this particular walking route is: It is inhabited by a tribe of young rebels, my kind of people.

Where my route turns south, if you go north instead, you'll be in the Lawrence Free State High School parking lot. Walk south across the school's parking lot and you'll meet up with my walking route which follows this little ditch, perhaps 50 yards in length – the "wetlands" where the cattails grow.

II

The Rebels: On warm days there's often a small gathering of highschoolers, sitting on the bridge structures, hidden from the sidewalk and roadway. Rumor has it that they're a clan of "dropouts" – kids doing just enough to get through school, but with no passion for any part of schooling … or, for that matter, for any part of life in general. It seems the school's administration has given up on them.

Face to face, they are what you'd expect: fiercely conforming to non-conformity, hair styled with unique cuts and dyed in wild colors, and their clothes from a decade or two back. Each rebel has some form of smoke in hand. At first they ignore Sue and I and keep to their lively chatterings as we pass; later they smile and say their howdies and have-a-good-days and then go back to their community enclave. They are always courteous, respectful, and outwardly happy – especially when we keep on walking by.

III

I Go A'callin': One day, walking alone, I decide I'll go a-callin, and so I edge myself off the stability of the sidewalk onto a steep-slope path of mud and trampled weeds, hold on as I round the bridge structure, and say, "Howdy, guys. How's it goin? My name's Randy and I pass this way ever so often. Thought I'd stop by and say howdy."

Lots of suspicious looks, and a few of downright alarm! Some hiding of smokes behind backs. A thick undercurrent of burning weed in the air. I ask, "I've been wondering: what kind of critters do you see down there in the cattails?"

Long pause, then the girl with the blue hair says: "Used to be a muskrat that'd swim around down here, but he hasn't been around for quite a while."

"How cool is that," I say, thinking how cool is it that she could tell a muskrat from a beaver or an otter, or from a whale for that matter. "How about red winged blackbirds?" I ask. "Maybe defending their territories."

About a week ago I'd watched a half-dozen or so red wings across the road, boasting their this-is-my-territory calls of "chonk la ree," "chonk la ree," and flitting from one cattail to another, then strutting their fluffed-winged colors from atop the cattail cobs. But the cattail patch over there is much more extensive, and it surrounds my Pond Two, a fairly nice-sized pond.

"No," from the more pensive one with half a head of crewcut, the other half a brush of bright orange, "but there's a red tail hawk that hangs out in the trees up by school, and we see him almost every day. He's pretty cool."

Hot dam, I'm thinking, they noticed my favorite correspondence bird. "Hey," I say, "be sure to talk nice to my friend the hawk. We're best of buddies, you know, and if you talk to him nice enough, he just may give you a tip or two that'll help make it a better day for you. Y'all have a good day." As I walk away, I carry with me a load of feeling a whole lot better about our drop-out, rebel kids. Once again, I hear the refrain in my head: "The Kids Are Gonna Be Alright."

IV

Bamboozled By Cattails: Nature has this strange habit of sneaking up on you and overwhelming each and every one of your many senses, oftentimes all of them at once. It's like being bamboozled by the goddess of bamboozlement.

Nature is not a cheapskate with Her bamboozling either; offerings are provided at frequent and unexpected intervals nearly every day. Bam! There's another one. Being bamboozled by nature is also free of charge – all you need to do is stop, look and learn, listen, and respect… but you do need to do those four.

I had one of those bamboozling moments on my walk the other day, a balmy November Saturday with a sharp breeze out of the south. I'd picked the route where I'd met the rebels a few weeks back. I hadn't been on this route for several days, even though it is one of my favorites.

Turning the corner, into the south wind and suddenly face to face with the noontime sun, the air is filled with a profusion of tiny dancing flakes, each glowing with its own glint of sunshine. The dance of little golden-whitish sun-flakes, the personalized aura of gold around each of them, the sun in my eyes and highlighting the whiteness of the flakes: I am disoriented (more than usual), discombobulated (more than usual), and filled with awe.

For a moment there I think the cancer fog has got me, taken more than just my breath away, and I am floating through the Milky Way of my final death-dance. I want to fall to my knees …

but I know that my cancer-wobbled legs might not be able to lift me upright again.

The possibility that the flakes might be blowing dust or maybe even snow crosses my chemo-mind. And finally I wonder about a sudden birthing of a cloud of lecherous little gnats, all with their poisonous stingers poised to get me.

From the spiritual to the sublime to the downright scary, all these "what-ifs" pass within seconds, after which I notice that I am still standing on the security of solid sidewalk. And so, with the stability of body-on-concrete, I can concentrate my mind on the real cause of the flutterings.

A closer look reveals that the little white thingies are seed parachutes, flaking off the cattails that live in the ditch that runs along the sidewalk, not more than 20 feet away.

Nothing but common cattail seeds. Nothing more; nothing less. My, but what a sight! I'd been bamboozled by one of the most common of all our plants, cattails. My, but wouldn't this be something for my rebel kids to see, to appreciate the wonder of it all, to perhaps be awestruck or maybe even gobsmacked enough that they would want to reconnect with Nature ... if not with the school and with the people who had left them behind.

V

Last Words: But this was a Saturday, the rebels had scattered to ports unknown. It's a shame they are not here to see the reality of what Nature has to offer. It's a shame because, even with the modern miracles of an entire library in every laptop device; even with a cinematic screen on every home's living room wall; and even with a small-screen view box and recording camera in every pocket ... you can't really capture the astonishment, nor the sublime of Nature.

To capture the true reality of Nature's essence, you need to sit in stillness, listen with an open heart, and consciously open every pore of your body – none of which is possible while receiving communion at the altar of artificial reality. So it is with a wistful heart that I capture the cattail display today ... all by myself.

Chapter 24 Interlude:
Cattails as Food, Shelter and Medicine

I

Cattails Naturally: In a short moment of Nature's bamboo-zling I had been treated to the birthing of thousands of little seeds, each of them coming from the womb of a brown cattail cob the size of a sausage, and each of them floating in the winds on its own cottony-thin sail. Those who have counted say there are 200,000 to 300,000 seeds per cob, and apparently all the cattails had decided to give birth on that day, just as I was walking by.

In addition to all the swirling flakes of cotton in the air, huge white clumps of seed flakes remained behind, still clinging to their momma plants. It's almost impossible to wrap your head around how all those seeds can come from thin little spikes of cattail womb, but cattails are one of the more common plants we can see almost anywhere there is even a spit of water for them to stand in.

Being one of our most common plants has given the cattail the opportunity to work itself into our food pantries and into our lives in many other ways ... while at the same time providing food, shelter and nesting sites for a host of wild critters.

All parts of the cattail are edible – from the roots to the young shoots to the growing leaves to the cobs and the pollen on the cobs. All you need do to feast on cattail is to know which part is palatable during which part of the year.

Roots (rhizomes) are edible pretty much year-round, eaten by gnawing on them like you would a radish. Young shoots are much like asparagus – with a bit more cooking needed to make them truly tender; young stems can be eaten raw or boiled; and the lower parts of the leaves can be used in salads. The young flowers can be boiled, covered in butter and eaten like corn on the cob. In mid-summer, the yellow pollen taken from the male flowers can be added to pancakes or mixed with flour to make delicious bread.

Cattail root systems are known for their ability to remove metals and other pollutants from water, but the plant also has medicinal value for people, including antiseptic properties to treat wounds, burns, stings, and bruises. Finally, cattail is being studied as a possible aid for cancer prevention.

But you don't have to eat the cattail or use it as medicine to enjoy its functionality. Temporary housing and floor mats can be made by weaving the durable leaves together. The cobs can be coated with grease or lard and lit to make into torches, and the cottony seeds have been used as insulation or padding. Save some of the pods, and since the cotton stays dry, they make good tender for starting fires.

It's not just for us humans that the cattail is useful; animals of all ilk – birds, muskrats, turtles, snakes, and fish -- use them for housing, protection, feeding areas, and food.

II

Last Words: My days of foraging in the wilds have been ousted with the incoming winds of cancer. But those rebels I met a few days back, why, I'm thinking they could learn a lot from Cattail.

Give them a shot at making floor mats or torches; let them taste of the year-round bounty of cattail – after learning when to pick it and how to fix it, of course; and for those interested, have them keep track of all the critters that move in and out of the cattails during one year's seasons.

And all the while they'd be working in nature, learning from nature, they would also be reaping the many proven benefits of being outdoors.[18] For the life of me, I can't think of a better way to help the next generation reunite its human spirit with the soul of Nature.

It wouldn't need to be everyone either – not everyone wants to be attuned to Nature. I'm thinking that if I could just get 12 rebels who want to learn about Nature, that would be enough. Just 12 rebels … and the baton could be passed on to the next generation.

18 Just a few of the many benefits of being outdoors include: 1) you will be happier and more relaxed 2) stress, cortisol levels, muscle tension and heart rates will be reduced, 3) self esteem will improve; 4) you will have more energy; 5) your vitamin D levels will go up – giving you protection against a load of bad guys, including: osteoporosis, depression, heart attacks, and even cancer. (All of these, of course, would be helpful for rebels of any age.)

Deer Teachers

Lesson #1: Years back, when we were still on the farm north of Lawrence, I got a wild hair to construct a simple, classical labyrinth by mowing the required three circuits into the prairie. Then, I took to walking my labyrinth, trying to draw the gods down to earth with me.

I went crazed for a while there and decided to walk my labyrinth at sunrise for a solid year. And so Pokey and I roused ourselves well before sunrise, trudged to the labyrinth, and I slow-walked to its center where I could watch the sunrise. Within minutes Pokey would be bored, and he'd be off, ranging the prairie, looking for excitement.

In the year I walked the labyrinth, I never got even one glimpse of the gods, but nature was willing to share some of her best with me: beautiful plants flourishing inside the labyrinth, including black eyed susan, bee balm, echinacea and purple prairie clover – plants that I'd never seen on the rest of our prairies; redtail hawks and vultures overhead, trying to see what the hell I was doing down there; a litter of cottontails born near the center of the labyrinth (and later moved – hopefully by the doe – to places more secure); a rafter of wild turkeys, hatched just off the labyrinth to the south; and the surprise of the year: a young fawn, still with bold white dots across her back.

I spotted the fawn one morning, lying motionless close enough to the southside path of the labyrinth that, with one step into the prairie, I could have bent down and touched her. Motionless is the key word here. Stock still, immobile, completely at-rest, cradled by the prairie grasses – even her breathing was soft and quiet, not a hint of fearful panting. Only her eyes moved slowly so she could follow me.

I watched to make sure Pokey wouldn't interfere with her reverie, but he was out and about, too busy sniffing out smells he could actually sense. A fawn's scent glands develop as it matures, so – along with the protective ability of its camouflage coloring – a young fawn will have no body odor that might attract predators. Plus, the mother doe typically keeps her visits short and often during the night … thus minimizing her odors in the area.

And so it was: fawn laid in a safe place while mother grazed the morning grasses; a newborn instructed to lay there and not move until mother comes back to fetch her. A first lesson, likely imprinted onto genes, that is crucial for the survival of the species. The fawn was there three or four mornings, then gone, off on her way to explore her own pathways to adulthood and to new seasons to come.

And to be sure, I was honored that mother had enough confidence in me that she put me in charge of babysitting, if for only a few mornings there.

II

Lesson #2: Sue and I are on a really nice walking trail whose entrance sits just behind Rock Chalk Recreation Center here in Lawrence, KS. It is a mostly woodsy trail, with a stretch that runs alongside Baldwin Creek (known by locals as Rattlesnake Creek).

We chat as we walk, but Sue goes suddenly (and uncharacteristically) quiet, stops abruptly, puts a hand out to stop me and points into the woods. There he is, a young fawn about half grown, standing there, nonchalantly staring at us. We exchange stares for what seems like an eternity. Then, all of a sudden, without a hint of warning, he wheels a 180 and bounds directly away from us, taking maybe six or seven huge deer leaps to cover 30 yards or so.

Just as suddenly as he bounded away from us, he hits the ground on his seventh leap. Like a deflated balloon he collapses all his body parts into a heap, and he becomes invisible to us, hidden behind a small tuft of grass and weeds.

All this activity is likely from directions given by his mother (unseen by us) – deer voices we humans can't hear. My guess is that one snort or huff from the doe told him to "Get your ass out of there. Now!" and a second kind of huff said, "Now lie down tight and make yourself into that ball that no one can see. Right now!"

For me the real wonderment here is not just the reactions, but the teachings that went before them. Teachings between mother and son, mother and daughter. I wonder how a human mother could possibly achieve results as dramatic as these. Or a football coach.

III

Lesson #3: So far as I know, Pokey never met up with the Fawn of the Labyrinth. But he did meet up with a few grown deer in his day, and one in particular taught both Pokey and the doe's fawn a lesson or two.

One afternoon Sue, Pokey, and I were out taking a walk in the woods, using a well-worn deer trail. As usual, Pokey was somewhere well out in front of us, taking on all comers … until he met up with a comer much too tough for him to handle.

We didn't see what happened, but we heard a loud huff, a stomp, and a wailing scream from Pokey. Then, around the corner comes Pokey, on a tear, tail between his legs, headed straight for me … where he then hides behind my legs, peeking out to see if he's been followed.

We laugh. Then, about 10 yards down the path we meet up with the troublemaker as we round a curve in the trail: a mother doe with a nearly-grown fawn at side. She huffs at us once, twice, stomps her front feet, huffs again, turns and trots off with fawn trailing behind.

Lessons learned: I will protect my baby … no matter how tough you think you are. Dogs and humans, listen up, this applies to you too. Little one, you better learn how this protection game is played, so you too will be able to take care of your offspring.

IV

Lesson #4: I am nature-walking with cancer, a few years after diagnosis. I've found a trail in a hideaway park that weaves several hundred yards through a thick cedar woods. The smell of cedar is delightful, enlightening, and has the aura of being spiritual. Plus, I like the scrunch, scrunch, scrunch sound I make as I trod along on the pea-gravel pathway.

As I enter the woods, the crows often follow along overhead so they can warn me that I am intruding on **their** turf. There's a resident red tailed hawk and a barred owl who, if I am early enough, one or the other of them may still be sitting on the dead tree limb, staring down at me.

And there is a herd of deer. Sometimes I catch a quick glimpse of just one deer; other times I'll see a small gathering of perhaps two or three does with fawns at side; once Sue and I spotted (and were able to take blurry pictures of) at least five does accompanied by their fawns as they drank from a runoff ditch.

And so, this has become a favorite walking path, and today I am scrunch, scrunch, scrunching along when I see her through a clearing in the trees: an adult doe, calmly grazing in a clearing about 40 or 50 yards away from the trail. I stop to see if I can get a better look.

As my last footstep registers its final scrunch, one short instant later, the doe's head jerks up from grazing, and she immediately focuses in my direction, ears up and alert. Apparently, it was OK for me to walk my way through her grazing grounds … so long as I kept moving along. But the instant I stopped moving along, I became a potential threat.

We watched each other for a few minutes, and I continued on my way. And she resumed grazing. The trail I am on makes a few turns here, and when I round the last one, I see her again, this time she is aimed in an entirely new direction – facing toward me. And I now see that she has a fawn alongside. The fawn is more interested in frolicking about and kicking up his heels than in grazing.

Mother doe seems disinterested in her fawn's antics, but she has placed him in a position where she can both keep him in sight **and** she can see where I am on the trail.

Lesson to fawn: Pay attention. At all times! Only rarely does danger come pre-announced, so you always need to be acutely aware of your surroundings. And finally, have your fun little one, I get that, but both you and that guy on the trail better also know that I will do whatever I need to do to protect you.

V

Last Words: I am continually amazed that, with all the distractions we humans have created for ourselves and then have allowed ourselves to be attuned to, we still have the ability to focus on anything natural.

Chapter 25 Interlude: Instincts

I

Dr. Spock: No mother deer has ever read The Common Sense Book of Baby and Child Care, Dr. Benjamin Spock's 1945 classic book whose central theme was that parents should be more nurturing and that mothers should be more responsive to the needs of their children.

Watching a doe with her fawn, it seems almost as if a mother deer (or perhaps a small herd of mother deer) wrote Spock's book for him long ago … perhaps even before books were being written. In today's psychological terms we might call the message of Spock's book the *maternal instinct,* written large onto the deer's brain.

But wait just a minute. There are a few things about instincts that are written in the fine print.

II

Instincts: An instinct is: a) a natural or inherent aptitude, impulse, or capacity; b) a largely inheritable and unalterable tendency of an organism to make a complex and specific response to environmental stimuli without involving reason; and c) a behavior that is mediated by reactions below the conscious level.

Scientists who study such things have come up with several lists of instincts that the human animal has. Compiling the lists from several scientists, you would have instinctive human-characteristics that include: anger, fear, panic, grief, pleasure/lust, play, shyness, curiosity, affection, sexuality, jealousy and envy, rivalry, sociability, sympathy, imitation, secretiveness, acquisitiveness, and creativity.

Notably absent from most (but not all) lists is the maternal instinct, and this is because most (but not all) scientists feel that the maternal instinct is a trait that we humans must learn. In other words, we are not naturally nurturing to our babies.

(Note: Humans who have a natural maternal instinct can be either male or female; it is not an instinct, whether learned or natural, limited to the female of our species.)

III

Instinct-less Humans: It seems that, once again, we humans are, in our approach to living our lives, a mite oddball in the overall realm of animals. We have basic drives (motivators), and we can be driven (some would suggest we are often driven by self-motivated institutions) to fulfill those drives. But we don't have many instincts (innate behaviors).

At least one scientist[19] thinks this is because most instincts are rigid, unchanging, and provoked by a simple stimulus; humans tend to be more flexible and adaptive.

IV

Last Words: Apparently in our rush to evolve our brainpower to gargantuan levels, a few natural instincts were left out. It seems that we have chosen, instead, to let our brains find out how to live naturally (including how-to practice the maternal instinct) … by reading about it, seeing it on TV or the small phone-screen, or listening to a lengthy how-to from someone pontificating from his or her personal pulpit.

Note to us, the brainy ones: We could all learn a lot just by watching Nature in action.

---

19 Gabriela A. Martorell, B.S., M.A., Ph.D., Professor of Psychology, Virginia Wesleyan University has written several books, including: *Life: The Essentials of Human Development; Child; and A Child's World: Infancy Through Adolescence*

Huddlers and Cuddlers

I

Introduction: I'm out and about, once again sauntering along one of my normal walking trails … when I see something moving up a hillside of short grass. But wait, did I really see it? Was it a shadow of some bird flying overhead? Or a snake-in-the-grass, slither-racing, trying to get away from my walking sticks? Or just the breeze moving the grasses? I stop, look harder, listen.

Then, I see another flash of shadow some 10 yards further up the hill. Dang. Whatever is moving in the grass is moving right along. I mark the spot and vow to re-check it later on.

A few days later I stealth-walk up to the site of the quick movements, camera in hand and ready for a quick snapshot. Yup. There they are: two or three little rodent-like creatures, fairy-like in looks and demeanor … running the hell away from my approach.

By the time I get the camera to my eye, they are well up the hill – they move so fast there's no telling if it's two or three little fairies … let alone trying to tell what species they really are.

I'm pretty sure they are (or rather, were) Kansas Prairie Voles, Microtus Ochrogaster, and pretty sure is good enough for me.

II

Airy Fairy Rodents: There are bunches of little fairy-like creatures that live in Kansas, including: moles, voles, chipmunks, field mice, pack rats, pocket gophers, kangaroo rats, and shrews. Other curious Kansas critters with underground lifestyles include the more-sizable groundhogs and prairie dogs.

Of the wee-ones listed above, all but the moles and shrews are fast-action rodents that skitter along pathways they have channeled through the grasses or down into the underground tunnels they have dug.

If you were a poet, a sage, a shaman, or of Irish descent, you might think that the pathways made by these wee, cute-faced, fairy-like rodents who travel and spend much of their time underground … were actually the pathways of fairies.

While it does take a quick eye to catch one of the fast-moving Lilliputian rodents in action, I see their trails in abundance along my daily walkways.

And, despite their ability to play hide-away most of the time, the more I've listened to the tales they have to tell, the more I've grown to like these fairy-like rodents *and* their stories.

III

Voles: Most of the vole's *diet* is herbivorous and consists of grasses, fruits and seeds, and the bark of young trees along with a wide array of underground munchies, including roots and rootlets, fungi and fungal mycelium, and the occasional nibble of tiny bugs, worms, bacteria and other microorganisms that exist in the soil.

Vole *trails* also offer byways along which they can grab quick bits of grass, maybe a bug or two. The trails are also highways the vole can use to make a quick getaway from any nearby predator – and predators are many: hawks, foxes, owls, coyotes, snakes ... and human lawn and garden lovers. As highways, the trails lead to one of many entrances to their underground burrows.

Almost all of the vole species spend a lot of their time in their *burrows*, only coming above ground for short times of food-searching, and our Kansas prairie voles are no exception. Their burrows are usually associated with patches of lush vegetation and can be immense undertakings, consisting of numerous surface entrances, extensively branched and interconnected tunnels and dead-end passages, and nesting and feeding chambers. Most vole burrowing is within 10 inches of the ground's surface.

IV

Huddlers and Cuddlers: But the big story of prairie voles is that, akin to only about 3% of all other mammals, they are monogamous – at least partially monogamous, in the sense that it is more social than sexual monogamy.

The specific genetics of the prairie vole creates a web of hormonal reactions that result in pair bonding, a character trait that does not exist in other voles. The male prairie vole enjoys a lifestyle of continuous contact with his female counterpart – they huddle and cuddle together for their entire lifetime. If the female vole dies, the male does not look for a new partner.

Apparently huddling and cuddling is relaxing for both partners – they often fall asleep as they huddle-cuddle. And the pair bonding is apparently more social than sexual – male voles may stray on occasion.

For many years all this was thought to be solely from interactions of those two hormones – oxytocin and vasopressin. But now – after some fancy gene editing eliminated the effects of oxytocin but did not edit-out the huddling and cuddling – it is clear that there's more to the story than just those two hormones. Perhaps an entire spider web of interconnections of all sorts of basic instincts, hormones, nerve pathways, organ systems, immune functions, and microbiota in all areas of the body.

Once again, Nature has the last at bat … and the nuance of Nature is far more complicated than any one at-bat solution. And so, we have a "fairy rodent," smaller than a baseball, with much to teach us about our own sexuality, about why we tend to be monogamous, about how huddling and cuddling can be so very satisfying.

V

Last Words: Well hell, Sue and I could have saved them the trouble of all that gene editing. After cancer came calling, I felt more and more like huddling and cuddling. Yeah, I know I know, the androgen deprivation therapies had something to do with my ability to pair bond without sex, but still …

There is a certain soothing, a relaxation into serenity, a comfort zone achieved that comes with huddling and cuddling – and I don't know (nor care) whether those feelings come along with a release of oxytocin or not.

Someday I plan to ask Sue if huddling and cuddling gives

her the same feelings I have – if I can ever catch her before she falls asleep in the midst of our huddle-cuddle.

Chapter 26 Interlude: Ruling Rodents

I

Introduction: OK, the mind has run rampant on me once again – thinking about the demise of mankind and what kind of creature would replace us (after the next mass extinction, say) … and what then?

The unbridled mind has created the following storyline:

II

Huge Rats: One storyline has it that rats the size of sheep will ultimately be our successors as rulers of the earth. This story relies on the fact that rats have extended their populations to almost every corner of the earth. And they ain't dumb – rats are said to be more intelligent than rabbits, gerbils and guinea pigs and maybe even as smart as dogs.

Put the two together – smarts and the ability to adapt to almost any environment – and rats seem to be mighty good candidates as earth-rulers.

The increased-size idea is the thinking that once an entire class of former earth-rulers (dinosaurs for example) are cut down by a mass extinction, the smaller ones that had been living underfoot (for example, the wee critters such as the *Purgatorius* that the rest of us mammals are supposed to have evolved from) can grow to much larger sizes.

Thus, back some 66 million years ago (or about 100,000 to 130,000 years after the K-Pg boundary)[20] there would have been a rat-sized, tree-dwelling, six-inch-long squirrel-like critter (*Purgatorius*) weighing in at 1.3 ounces … that would eventually evolve into an animal the size we human mammals have become and on up to today's largest mammal, the Antarctic blue whale that

---

20 The K-Pg boundary marks the end of the Cretaceous Period, the last of the Mesozoic era, and marks the beginning of the Paleogene Period.

weighs in at up to 400,000 pounds (approximately 33 elephants) and reaches up to 98 feet in length.

III

Growing Brains: The story of rats the size of sheep has its appeal, but my thinking has added an addendum to it:

We humans had an intense surge of brain growth – both brain size and creative ability took an enormous jump about 40,000 years ago. The suddenness of the growth surge defies all ideas of normal evolution, so something profound must have happened.

One theory has it that this profundity came about because humanoids were grazing on mushrooms, especially psychedelic ones such as psilocybin.[21] The blast of neuronal tripping that ensued allowed humans the ability to expand their thoughts, and thus their brains grew. And their creative capacities soared.

Now, snubbing the stuffy old scientists, let's transfer this theory into the voles, our underground fairy rodents – all of whom spend their lifetimes literally swimming in a seabed of fungal mycelium. How long will it take them to randomly gnaw on enough of the psychedelic mycelium to begin to have mind-expanding journeys that eventually take them into realms where their brains are allowed to grow?

Who knows how long this might take? Only the underground shadow can tell us.

But I like to think the likelihood (however small) could still remain that underground fairy rodents will eventually develop expanded brains and brain capacities, maybe becoming as smart as we think we are.

And remember, the voles have developed the art of huddling and cuddling – leading to more a cooperative union of spirits … as opposed to our human way of trying to become the most competitive bastards we can possibly muster.

And when the next mass extinction comes along, the voles

---

21 This theory, sometimes referred to as the Stoned Ape Theory, was proposed by Terrence McKenna in his 1992 book Food of the Gods which used evidence largely based on studies by Roland L. Fischer's work from the 1960s and 1970s. Most scientists nowadays have rejected the theory, arguing that McKenna misinterpreted Fischer's works. But what the hey – any story about a stoned ape sounds like a rollicking good fairy tale to me.

could grow in size as well as enhancing their smarts. And think about it: they have already adapted to our human-populated areas and to the style of living we have achieved. Give them some added size along with added smarts and cooperative spirits, and they could take over our abandoned houses, learn to drive our cars, and then begin to live the life of luxury we now enjoy.

Think about it. But maybe put a bridle on your thinking … so you can rein it in before it runs away with you.

IV

Last Words: If we ever plan to understand what the earth is really about, we will need to understand its underground components – where 70% of all life occurs. And we would do well to think about what might lie ahead for you and me and the rest of our species – a future we might be able to glean from listening to the stories today's underground critters can tell us.

Skin of the Earth

I

Introduction: It's springtime and I'm sauntering … with a purpose. My purpose today is to see some of my long-time buddies, and right away I'm rewarded: my friends, the birds, are everywhere active. Robins hop-hop-hopping along, pacing the lawns, looking for earthworms, then flying back and forth, ground to tree-nest, to feed their new brood. Doves with their hauntingly-mournful cooing. Grackles cackling at each other. An occasional Cardinal or Blue Jay showing off their colors, and lots and lots of LGBs (Little Grey Birds) flitting hither thither and yon.

Rabbits are also present in profusion. Nibbling on the freshly mown lawns. Watching me nervously. All sizes of rabbits – evidence that the first batch of kits has been kicked out of the warren, and the doe is out and about, fattening up for the next litter.[22]

These are the buddies I see, but a whole class of buddies – the medicinal weeds – are nowhere to be seen … at least on this first part of my trek that covers about a half-mile. I am walking a vast expanse of weed desert, front lawns overgrown with bright-green, well-manicured (and well-weeded) grass.

Amazingly, I don't even see one yellow-topped dandelion for the full half-mile. Until I turn the corner that leads onto the De-Victor Loop, a popular Lawrence trail for bird watching, hiking and running.

II

Medicinal Weeds: On the DeVictor Loop's first part I will be walking alongside a wild streambed, and looking into the back

---

22 Young rabbits disperse from the nest at 15-20 days old. By three weeks of age the pint-sized young'uns are on their own in the wild and no longer require a mother's care. The Eastern Cottontails are indigenous to Kansas, and an adult will weigh in at about 2 to 3 pounds, maybe up to 4 pounds for one overfed on lawn grasses.

yards of those well-lawned houses that adorned the first part of my walk.

Enter the Loop and the scenery immediately changes – the medicinal weeds (and wild edibles) are in abundance. Dande-lions of course, and also plantain, burdock, and mullein for my medicine chest; a small patch of Chenopodium (aka: goose foot) for a breakfast frittata; and lots of common milkweed to keep the butterflies happy.

About 100 yards into the DeVictor and you make a sharp right turn onto a corridor that rests atop an underground gas pipeline easement. You are now walking between the backyards of suburban houses on both sides of the easement, the limits of the easement marked by the backyard fences of the homes.

The easement walkway becomes a mix of manicured lawns, weedy lawns and patches of mostly-weeds ... which then results in a beautiful array of medicinal weeds here and there, scattered throughout. Interestingly, on this section you can see into most, but not all, of the backyards, and many of them have lush gar-dens – both vegetable and flowering gardens. The gardens are often lovely … but typically lack even one medicinal weed.

The last section of this walk is along another section of suburb, and the lawns are noticeably different: some (like those of the first part of my walk) have zero weeds; others a more scattering of dandelion and perhaps plantain and/or mullein. One lawn is almost covered in yellow – dandelions in full bloom … and I'm thinking that particular lawn may be a mite over-medicated.

III

Skins: You and I and the creatures of the earth walk on the skin of a very alive organism – our Earth Mother. As philoso-phers attempt to rough-sketch the boundaries of the Self, so too do cartographers attempt to draw the lines that separate land from water, hill from vale, friend from foe.

Having established their boundaries, it is time for the visual artists to take over. Topographers use different colors to indi-cate land elevations and the general lay of the land; the land's coverings – water, forest, prairie, and population densities; other colors to indicate where natural pathways (waterways, for example) and man-made pathways (such as highways and rail-roads) have been built.

Anatomy artists use a similar color-coded technique to separate epidermis from dermis and then to separate these skin structures from more inner organs and the pathways that connect the organs.

Even the physical layout of skin-of-man and skin-of-earth appears much the same.

Our skin is: 1) an epidermal outer layer of dead and dying cells that faces the outside world and tells us the story our environment brings us today; 2) this outside story is then relayed via nerves of the inner layer of dermal skin to pathways that offer sensate inputs to our organs and their inner systems as well as providing us with proprioception info that helps keep us upright; 3) a porous covering, pin-pricked with tiny tunnels that exude sweat and scents that mark us as human; 4) forested with hair rooted in the nutrient-rich dermis and even deeper; 5) home to populations of microbiota that offer a way of communication – between the outside world and the inner immune systems. And finally, 6) our skin comes in a variety of colors … a spectrum of colors that give us reason to celebrate the diversity of our humanity.

Skin of the Earth: Leaf debris and grass clippings and wind-blown sands provide an initially-protective skin for Mother Earth. This "skin of the earth" is then transformed into the top-soil which becomes nutrient and nerve center … which ultimately acts as the creator of all the foods that feed us.

Mother Earth's skin is also porous, with pores that range in size from the tiny seeping springs that then go on to create huge rivers … to the already-huge volcanic openings that spew gasses and minerals from well-below. The earth's skin, much like our skin, has many fingers extended outward so it can sense its environment – an environment that extends upward from the velveteen ground-hugging mosses up to the tip-tops of the giant sequoias.

IV

The Underground/Dermis: Scientists tell us that about 70% of all life on earth is subterranean – the **underground** is quite literally alive – teeming with living organisms: bacteria, archaea, fungi and fungi-like actinomycetes, algae, and protozoa. These microscopic entities are in constant interaction with a wide variety of larger soil fauna which spend all or part of their life underground: mites, nematodes, earthworms, ants, and insects.

Much of the living underground structure is composed of bulbs, roots, rootlets, and root hairs, randomly woven together with a network of fungal threads or hyphae (mycelium) to form a dense tapestry of communicating threads of life. It is likely that the mycelium compose the life-form with the largest total mass of living organism on earth,

And then, all of these underground entities are in constant intercourse with the even larger organisms – including the moles, voles, and the rest of the burrowing rodents.

The *dermal layer of human skin* makes up 90% of skin's thickness. This middle layer of skin has collagen and elastin which help make the skin strong, resilient, and flexible. The dermis houses the sweat glands, hair, hair follicles, muscles, sensory neurons, and blood and lymph vessels. All these dermal entities are in constant intercourse with the even larger organs and organ systems deep within our bodies.

V

Last Words: And so, the earth connects with the outer world through its outer skin … and we connect to our outer world through our skin.

Now, wouldn't you think it would be wise for us to try to understand how to connect our two skins – the earth's and ours – in a natural and healthy manner … instead of trying to obliterate the connections with a constant mowing, scraping, plowing and digging into it. And, on the other hand, scrubbing and abrading our skin with soaps loaded with often-toxic chemicals, dowsing our bodies with flowery-smelling skin lotions, and treating every nick and scrape with antibiotics that kill everything in their path … and referring to this as "skin care."

One can only hope that, as we mature into a species with an understanding for the importance of our interconnections between our Selves and Nature, we will finally learn how to view both skins – the skin of Mother Earth and our own skin – as sacred objects, worthy of honor and respect.

Perhaps then we will be able to tell a new story of creation, a story of health and healing – beginning from the outside and working its way in … or would that be beginning from the inside and working its way out?

Chapter 27 Interlude: Lymphatics

I

Lymphatics: Swimming along through the layers of skin, flowing deep into internal body parts, and wrapping around the internal surface of the gastrointestinal and respiratory tracts is a special network of capillaries known as the lymphatic system.

This network of veins and arteries interconnects with some 400 to 800 bulb-like lumps of tissue (lymph nodes) whose jobs include: 1) transporting immune information across all body systems; 2) filtering incoming lymph fluids and screening out invading germs they might carry; and 3) playing a role in malignancy (such as my prostate cancer).

Lymph nodes are concentrated in the neck, under-arms, chest, belly, and groin … and scattered throughout the rest of the body. A typical lymph node is barely palpable when in its healthy state; when infected or infiltrated with cancer cells, it can balloon to huge proportions – thus damming up the normal flow of lymph fluid.

II

Lymphedema: When lymph can't flow along at its normal rate, it escapes its veins and accumulates in pools of squishy fluids – referred to as lymphedema. Cancer is a relatively common cause of lymphedema … but there's an even more-insidious cause: radiation therapy meant to cure the cancer.

In my case, after the first go-around with chemo-therapy, my rogue cancer cells eventually decided to infiltrate my pelvic lymph nodes and cause them to grow in response – which made taking a dump an hour-long grunt-filled challenge. At best.

My oncologist advised radiation therapy. And the radiologist, a charming young man, agreed, saying he thought he could, by zapping the offending nodes into oblivion, free up my sewage systems for at least six months or more.

Having spent much of the past several weeks sitting on the John, sweating and grunting, I thought radiation sounded like a better plan. But once again, I forgot to read the fine print.

Turns out that burning the nodes and their interconnecting capillaries into oblivion wreaks havoc on the lymph system's normal functioning. A certain percentage of radiation patients develop lymphedema – initially around the area of radiation; later on perhaps throughout the body.

In my case my legs got puffy with the edema, then my scrotum began to swell. And swell, and swell. Until it is now the size of a nice, juicy grapefruit. My oncologist tells me she has nothing for my condition … unless I want to go through another round of chemo.

My oncologist sends me to the urologist who reiterates: "Nothing I can do for you. Maybe surgery, but that's often not too good. Liposuction sometimes works, but usually for a short time only. The edema tends to gravitate to the lowest body part, and in your case the scrotum and your legs are the lowest parts of body below where they did the radiation. In some people the scrotum gets huge."

I looked it up: Lymphedema as a result of pelvic radiation can create scrotums bigger than cantaloupes … or even watermelons. (By then you'd likely be a goner, but one supposes, could you live that long, the scrotum would eventually grow into weather-balloon size. My what a sight that would be to behold.)

The fine print also tells me that, along with the lymphedema, severe skin infections often develop – something more for me to worry about.

As we are leaving the urologist's office, he adds one more thought: "Remember, the edema will tend to develop in areas where gravity takes it. I'm not so sure exercise is a great option; maybe bed rest would be best for now." (And, I'm thinking: "Or standing on my head for the rest of my life.")

III

My Response: And so, I go to a massage therapist who specializes in lymph massage, and I learn how to massage at least some of the lymph into areas where my lymph system is still intact. And for tea-time I sip on lymph cleansing herbs such as: burdock, dandelion, red clover, and cleavers. And I say "screw you " to bed rest, and try to keep up my walking routine … while toting a few extra pounds bound up in my compression shorts, between my legs.

IV

Last Words: Seems to me just another case of a system/institution (oncology medicine) running amok … and in this case, using my scrotum as the ultimate punching bag. All in the name of giving me a few extra months of life … no matter the cost. A system working under the assumption that I – like most cancer patients in our culture – want to stay alive as long as possible … no matter the cost. All this without ever asking *me* what *I* really want – to do, to have, to be.

Kansas Rocks

I

Creating Rock: Several forms of creation have been used to bring us the three species of rocks we commonly see here in Kansas – limestone, flint, and Siouan Quartzite.

Limestone: Most of Kansas sits atop what was once an inland sea – a mostly shallow ocean of water that extended from the Gulf of Mexico through the U.S. and Canada meeting with the Arctic Ocean. For millions of years, huge sea creatures swam in the waters over Kansas – 59 foot-long reptiles, 33 foot-long shell-eating sharks, and the largest ever bony fish, the Xiphactinus. Tiny invertebrate and shelled critters – mollusks, plankton, and squid-like creatures – swam alongside their spooky-looking cousins.

As the masses of sea-swimmers died, they left behind layers of calcium. Then, this calcium from living bone and shell – under the pressure of the waters above and being worked by the ebb and flow of the varying levels of the sea – created layer upon layer of limestone. Additionally, a layer of mud – hardened into shale – often separates limestone layers, and these rocky layers can easily be seen alongside cuts in Kansas roads. The abundance of fossils imprinted into the rock formed millions of years ago make the roadside layers ideal hunting grounds for paleontologists, both amateur and professional.

Flint is created as if by morula growth within the womb of shell and bone.

I am told that technically "chert" is the correct term for the form of flint rock found around here in the Flint Hills. Geologists consider chert as a lesser quality flint, a type of flint that – because it is made under lesser pressure from above than true flint – is slightly softer than "true" flint.

Almost anywhere in the pastured Flint Hills you can walk the hills and find chunks of chert, varying in size from what you can hold in the palm of your hand up to huge boulders.

Siouan Quartzite: Several years back Sue and I drove the 300-plus miles to Sioux Falls, South Dakota. After we'd settled into the motel, we became tourists and visited Falls Park, a site where, for eons, the Big Sioux River has cascaded over a bed of enduring Quartzite, eventually creating a 100-foot-high water-fall.

The red boulders that frame the waterfall are a part of over 6,000 square miles of Sioux Quartzite that spreads over portions of South Dakota, Minnesota, and Iowa, and tall outcroppings of the rock formations can be spotted across the countryside. It is these outcroppings of red rock far to the north of us that have provided the Siouan Quartzite rocks and boulders that are scattered over the prairies of Kansas.

Our metamorphic red rocks were born some 1.6 billion years ago, the result of nature combining microscopic bits of several different kinds of rock crystals into a goo that was then subjected to millions of years of water pressure from the inland sea that divided North America at the time. The resultant rock – our Siouan Quartzite – is hard enough to spark when struck with steel and was, for a time, used for constructing buildings and as paving bricks.

Even more impressive than their origin story is how our red rocks got to Kansas – propelled here during the Ice Age glaciations, hundreds of thousands of years ago.

I have a difficult time conjuring what a sheet of ice would look like: a wall of frozen water hundreds of feet high, creeping along, inches at a time … crawling over the ground as the millennial rhythms of the climate and the breath of the seasons and the pulse of night and day worked to edge them along.

Red boulders and rocks and rock rubble, somehow pushed along or picked up and carried by those ice sheets – our gift from the climate gods and from an expanse of rock-lands born far to the north. For the life of me, I can't see how any of this was created without some form of spirit helping. Most certainly this creation did not come from human hands.

II

Working Stone: Many of the individual prairie tribes had their arrowhead artisan, the tribal *flint knapper.* According to area archeologists, the local tribe's knapper often sat atop a ridge of one of the Flint Hills just west of Lawrence, Kansas – working with rocks. His job was to make tools – arrowheads, fleshing knives, hide scrapers and more – out of the natural flint/chert found as hard rock deposits within the softer limestone of the hills.

While the tribal flint knapper was busily making tools from flint, his job was also to be a lookout – noting where game was, watching for migrating bison herds, alert for enemy approach. All this an integral part of tribal life, and if you know what you're looking for, you can still find the spot where the flint knapper sat, perhaps thousands of years ago, leaving his flint shards and the rubble of his mistakes behind.

Making Flint Tools: I have watched as arrowheads are being made. It looks easy. Hold a hard rock in one hand and forcefully thunk it onto a chunk of flint that's about the size of a softball or maybe a bowling ball, striking along the fracture lines of the flint.

The idea is to make smaller stones from larger ones by pounding the flint-chunk until it eventually shatters at its edges, cleaved along those natural fracture lines within the rock. The knapper hopes the flint-chunk will yield, after all that pounding, a shard of hard rock flint, flatter than the original chunk. Hopefully the shard will be one of about arrowhead or knife size.

That piece of flint is then worked into edges that are sharp as the steel of a knife blade. Deer or elk antlers are typically used for this stage, and the idea is to press antler into hard rock until the rock yields and gives up a small flake of rock … leaving a sharp edge behind as the beginnings of an arrowhead or a fleshing tool or a knife.

III

Me the Knapper: All this looks easy enough when you're watching an expert at work, and in fact, there are entire books on the subject. You can even join one of the many clubs located across the country where you can learn how to make arrowheads alongside other flint knappers.

I've tried my hand at flint knapping: My hand-held hard-rock smacks the chunk of flint I've picked from the prairie. Nothing. Repeat. Nothing. Repeat, harder. Nothing. Swing rock from shoulder height. Nothing but clunk, reverberating back up to and through the shoulder.

After several minutes of this, I give up and go get a hammer. Swing hammer at flint rock. Nothing. Swing harder. Nothing. Go for a bigger hammer. Nothing. Swing even bigger hammer, now a post-driving maul. Nothing. Swing again from overhead. Finally, finally something happens – the flint shatters into hundreds of tiny fragments and a small pile of flint dust.

Had I been the tribal knapper, these could have been the flint rubble piles you can still find atop our Flint Hills – work sites from days gone by. And I most certainly would not have lasted long as the tribal tool maker. It obviously takes an artisan, a person willing to read and listen to the flint … as the rock explains how and where the arrowhead exists within. I am not that artisan.

IV

Rock Art: Artists who work with rock, and especially Indigenous sculptors, often talk of how their task is to give birth to what the rock contains within. They simply carve into the stone until that art form is revealed to the rest of us. And so, perhaps a question we commoners should ask the rock-workers is: Do all rocks contain things – tools, art forms, entire representations of human bodies (or the bodies of other beings), and more – entities that most of us cannot see.

V

Rock Spirits: Thinking of stones and spirituality, I am reminded of a pathology lesson reinforced by the story told by our professor, a story about *osteo petrosis*, a rare hereditary disease also known as "stone bone" and "marble bone." *Osteo petrosis* is a hardening of bone where bones thicken and become as hard as rock, eventually leading to death. (*Osteo petrosis* should not be confused with osteoporosis, a disease that often occurs with age and that results in a softening of bones due to calcium loss.)

"Remember it this way class," our professor pointed out, "St. Peter's Basilica was built on solid rock: *Osteo* is Latin for bone; *petrosis* derives from St. Peter and his Basilica … set on rock.

St. Peter's Basilica is more than built on rock; it is made of rock. And artworks carved from rock that are meant to connect you to the spiritual realm reside within.

VI

Last Words: I find it awesome that all things of nature – from the inanimate to the animate – have the capacity to provide us with functional "tools" … and to satisfy some of our spiritual needs.

Chapter 28 Interlude: Listening to Rocks

I

My **Rock:** I have a rock a little bit bigger than a softball that sits in my office in a place of respect. I have set it there because it has the uncanny ability to speak to me in ways I can understand. It's true that I need to drum and smudge myself into a state of mind where I am able to shuck the mind-poisoning that too much scientism-schooling has left me with, but when I am listening to it just so, that rock can speak in ways both intelligible and informative.

This is my rock's story:

It is early 1980's, and I am nearly finished with my PhD studies when I decide to enroll in a weekend workshop, given by Sandra Ingerman.[23] The workshop is advertised to offer some of the basic teachings of shamanism, and I need a break from the rigors of graduate school, trying to learn reams and reams of un-

23 Sandra Ingerman is an award-winning author of 12 books and presenter of 8 audio programs produced by Sounds True. She is a world-renowned teacher of shamanism and has been teaching for close to 40 years. Sandra is recognized for bringing ancient cross-cultural healing methods into our modern culture addressing the needs of our time, especially those concerning the environment.

related factoid data-bits. Out of the books and back to the spirit of nature, so to speak.

My plan is to drive to the workshop site south of Kansas City, and several of us will camp out on the site. However, as usual, I am running late. If I don't hurry, I will have to put my tent up in the dark. I am speeding down what is now called The Road To Oz Highway, a curvy two-lane road, heading south out of Wamego. The Road To Oz Highway seems like a fitting moniker for the path I am taking.

As I drive, I'm taking stock of what I have loaded into the pickup to take along: tent, sleeping bag, vittles for two days, water, change of clothes, and … ooops.

I now remember that, according to directions in the workshop's brochure, we were supposed to bring along a rock, about softball or cantaloupe sized. The lesson will supposedly be something about listening to what a rock can tell you. Maybe if I wasn't such a rock-head, I would have remembered to have one with me. Damn. Well, maybe I can find one at the campsite, I'm thinking … when, rounding a corner, driving dangerously fast, I see a gleam. A glistening in the sun as if the sun itself were down there in the ditch.

I slam on the brakes, quick stop, and collect the stone. The perfect rock for me – it's one of the Sioux Quartzite stones. This area south of Wamego has entire hillsides dotted with these stones, varying in size from boulders to the baby-sized one I've just found.

And so, me and my rock will attend the workshop together. Once there and during one of the sessions of the workshop, we learn a technique that directs me to think of a question I want to ask the rock. Then, with my question in mind, I look at four surfaces of the rock and read four images that appear to me on each side. I write down the images seen on the rock and have a partner verify that she also sees what I think I see (and that I'm not just BS-ing). From the visions, I am to make a story that should answer my question.

"Yeah right," I'm thinking. So, I do as a good little workshop attendee would do, report my story (that makes absolutely no sense to me), and take my rock home with me … along with a mountain-sized load of skepticism.

II

The Job Interview: Several months after the workshop, I am gearing up for a job interview in Dallas, and I'm thinking, what the hell, let's give the rock a shot. So, I decide to ask my rock: "What will happen to me on this job interview trip?" It'll be me and the rock, trying to conjure what lies before me, possibly for the rest of my life.

Here's what I see (all of these confirmed by Sue, my very indulgent wife): Several turtles (turtles?); a few bicycles (bicycles?); a white-capped mountain (Snow? In Dallas?); the compelling image of what looks to be some sort of female African tribal warrior figure, complete with a flowing Rasta-like hair style and carrying a shield (what???); a bear (in Dallas?); several pairs of eyeglasses; and an airplane.

Yeah, well, I'll be taking an airplane to get there, and I'm guessing almost everyone working there will be wearing eyeglasses – so, two for … how many? None of this makes a damned bit of sense to me, but I write it all down in my journal and finish packing for the trip.

My first interview is with one of the veterinarians who works there, and I am ushered into her office. After a few minutes' wait, in walks a beautiful black lady with shoulder-length Rasta-style hair braids, wearing a wildly-colored traditional dress and carrying a clipboard. I stand to shake her hand, my knees go weak, and I must sit down. My rock's warrior lady has appeared – with a clipboard shield.

Next stop: the boss' office. As I wait for him, I notice his bike parked along the wall. (I'll be damned!) I look at the framed map on the wall above the bike, and there's a white-capped mountain beside a pond that is circled by bike trails. (I'll be double damned!) When the boss arrives, wearing eyeglasses, I ask about the white-capped mountain, and he explains that it's really white sand, not snow. "It's beside one of the favorite bike trails in Dallas," he adds. "I try to ride on it whenever I can."

Lunch time: we drive past a small creek, and as we cross a bridge over the creek, I notice several turtles nonchalantly sunning on rocks. We dine at the Turtle Creek Inn. I am beginning to suspend disbelief in rock teachings.

After a day of interviews, I board the plane to take me back to Kansas City and pull out my journal to see how my rock performed. Well, I'll be damned. My rock got it right, damned near everything – all but one: the bear.

I smugly relax into my seat, thinking, The Rock ain't so smart after all. I open the flight magazine, leaf through it until... I am stopped dead by a vodka ad – using an attack bear, leaping out from the page, trying to scare me into buying their product. OK, disbelief is now totally suspended.

III

Last Words: So, were you to ask me if rocks have spirit, spiritual qualities, I'd have to say "yes, indeed. At least for me."

And then there's one of my favorite-of-all-times poems, "Tide," written by the uncle of one of our sons-in-law, H. C. Palmer—which I guess makes him a member of our extended family.

TIDE

H.C. Palmer

My father believed the bedrock beneath our ranch –
      once an immense sea –
was still alive, that natural rhythms persisted
      in its sluggish consolidation.
He taught me to listen for echoes of breaking surf,
      but I couldn't hear them –
even at night with the wind quiet and my ear pressed
      to an outcropping.
He believed the gravitational pull of a full perigee
      moon could still move
the old limestone. He called it land tide. I thought
      that too, improbable
until one night the moon rose so full of light we could
      have counted the calves
in our pasture. Then, when its bottom edge caught
      the crest of a hill,
and just as I felt the prairie lift and inch sideways
      beneath my feet,
he said. There. That's it.

I have never recovered from that night, or the weight of his
hand on my shoulder.[24]

---

24 Prior to a career in internal medicine, Dr. H.C. Palmer was a battalion surgeon in the American War in Vietnam. He has also been a cattle rancher and now a poet. Before Vietnam, H.C. played football and ran track for the KU Jayhawks, and Sue and I know him as the uncle of one of our sons-in-law. This poem is from his book of poems: *Feet of the Messenger,* © 2017, BkMk Press.

Cottonwood, *Populus spp.*

I

Introduction: Our bed's headboard fits snuggly up against the north wall of our bedroom. Our bedroom has a spacious window facing west, and the window looks out onto another apartment complex below. Sue insists on open windows; our blinds and curtains are almost never closed … including at night. The east end of the apartment complex below us and to our west is lined with cottonwoods – they are there because there's a small ditch that catches runoff from the line of parking garages.

Their placement makes them the ideal figureheads for sending shadow images onto our east bedroom wall, catching the night lights of the apartments. I know when the winds blow – the cottonwood shadows are moving, oftentimes briskly moving about. I know when the seasons are changing: summertime the shadows are heavy with leaves; wintertime only the bare limbs are shadowed.

Sometimes our east bedroom wall is an eerie shadow of suspense; most times though I welcome my contact with the outdoors … a contact I can make without leaving the comfort of my covers.

II

Our Cottonwoods: Our cottonwoods to the west are also a birder's delight. Most of the birds we see during the day use them as a hop-off spot during their travels north and south. We watch as the goldfinches land there, and the crows, robins, bluebirds, bluejays, sparrows, mourning doves, grackles, and of course, the starlings that are using the nooks and crannies of our apartment roof as their nesting sites. Cottonwood leaves and branches offer a haven for all sorts of bugs, butterflies, and beetles, and at least one squirrel has his summertime drey stuck in the fork of one of the tree's branches.

In addition to the trees outside our west windows, sitting on our deck, looking out into the neighborhood's view-scape we can spot the cottonwoods among the other trees. They are especially easy to spot in the fall – they are the first trees to change colors, from green into a bright yellow-gold. You can bet that wherever you see a cottonwood there will be a source of water under its roots.

III

The Spirit of Cottonwood: In the summer and fall, when they are in full leaf, the cottonwoods become more than mere water indicators; they are a source of inspiration, almost spiritual in quality. This should come as no big surprise. In addition to being practical structures, trees have always had that air of the spiritual. Consider the Christian Christmas tree, the Buddhist Bodhi tree, the sacred oak of the Celts, and the African Baobab, among others.

But the cottonwood is specially constructed to create a spiritual feel. Their leaves are heart-shaped and aerodynamically constructed to catch the winds. Our Kansas winds are legendary, so there is an almost constant rattling and whispering of cottonwood leaves in the winds hereabout.

As the cottonwood leaves catch the ever-constant winds, they also reflect the sunlight and moonlight. And so, there is that rattling of leaf against leaf, coupled with the glittering of leaf-reflected lights. It is no wonder that the Native Americans sat under the cottonwoods so they could listen as the gods spoke to them – I have done this myself.

Then there's that thing about stars and cottonwoods. Take a twig of the cottonwood, snap it just right, and voila there's a star shape hidden within. One more reason to think of the heavens – while snapping cottonwood twigs … just for the hell of it.

IV

Cottonwood Guideposts: Here in Kansas, it is flat as far as you can see. Mountains are not a part of the lay of the land – but the cottonwoods are.

Think about the frontierswoman, jouncing along in her Prairie Schooner, trying to visualize where the trail is taking her family... and when she and her family and the oxen will be able to take in their next drink of spring water. Or consider the trapper searching for his next beaver colony, knowing that beaver will be his door to the prosperity he has traveled all the way from Europe to make his own. On a nearly treeless prairie, flat as a soda cracker, an empty horizon is not much help for giving directions. Cottonwood to the rescue.

A fully grown cottonwood can stand 70 to 100 feet tall, and on flat ground you can spot one that is about 10 to 12 miles away – about the distance a covered wagon could travel in half a day. And so, you pack up and get moving in the morning, and with good luck, you'll be able to see where you'll be eating lunch and letting the oxen rest and feed – the tops of the cottonwood will be your guidepost as you move along. Then the next cottonwood will act as shepherd, helping guide you to your nighttime stopping place or to the place where you'll be able to make a safe crossing at a creek or river.

Some of these cottonwood stopping places still have the tree in place, oftentimes a tree so huge by now that it would take four or five adult arm-spans to try to encircle it for a group hug. One of those trees exists just south of Lawrence, still standing where the Oregon Trail crossed the Wakarusa River.

V

Nurturing Cottonwood: Cottonwood spreads her seed on the wind, and wind is a constant factor of the prairie. Seeds blow on a cottony parachute; those that come to rest on muddy soil root quickly and even more quickly sprout into seedlings. These seedlings provide the structural bed that stabilizes the riparian shoreline of streams, rivers, and ponds.

It's a mutual payback: Torrents of water from intense prairie thunderstorms leave rivulets of water that roam the prairie randomly; these erosion-producing rivulets are contained into the streams and rivers that the roots of cottonwood have woven into shoreline firmament. The contained river, in turn, provides water for the growth of the cottonwood.

And so, cottonwood tames the prairie, and in turn the tamed prairie feeds the cottonwood. And while this is the backstory of cottonwood and prairie, the tree offers us much more.

Cottonwood leaves and bark are rich sources of protein and can be used for livestock feed when other sources are not available. The inner bark contains a healthy mix of compounds, including flavonoids, polyphenols, and salicin -- a combination which provides a potent brew for easing pain and inflammation and killing bacteria. The wood of the cottonwood, while soft, is a decent source of lumber for buildings and fences. And as we've seen, the tree's foliage is a sanctuary for all sorts of critters.

VI

Nature Always Bats Last: Finally, cottonwood is a tough old geezer, but while she is tough enough to resist drought and fires common on the prairie, she isn't one to stick around forever. The typical cottonwood reaches her peak size in about a hundred years, and then she begins to fall apart. As her limbs break off, the tree's decaying infrastructure makes for myriad cracks and crevices in her trunk … which provide even more habitat for critters looking for a tree home.

But a tree falling apart and losing its huge limbs is not the best tree to plant next to your house or garage. Not content to drop their limbs on your buildings (and on the occasional person who happens to be walking below), a cottonwood likes to push up its roots, potentially lining your yard with trip-over obstacles … or maybe even uprooting the corner of your house. Plus, those seeds that fly off on their cottony parachutes every spring – each female tree able to produce up to 25 million seeds each year – can wreak havoc on drains, gutters, and landscapes.

VII

Last Words: And so, we, being the true synanthropes here – the ones who have intruded into the lives of cottonwoods and their ability to be mutually beneficial to the prairie and the wild species living on it – perhaps we should rethink our intense desire to have dominion over all of Nature. Perhaps a better approach might be to learn how to live within the boundaries and parameters set by wild nature … long before we were here.

Chapter 29 Interlude: Cottonwoods

I

Cottonwood Recap: And so, we see that cottonwood is designed to have many functions and purposes – both tangible and transcendent. As stewards of Nature, it is now our responsibility to apply these attributes with respect.

II

Stop, Look & Learn, Listen, Respect: It's easy to walk right by a cottonwood and not even notice her/him. She/he is, after all, just a tree. And even on the Kansas prairie where there aren't a lot of trees, there are enough of them that they often become invisible. The trick, as a trickster, is to make those trees pop out of the background noises of civilization.

Stop. Nature has a magical way of erasing those annoying and unnecessary twitterings of the mind … but you may need to stop and focus to get the eraser to work. With a being as monumental as an adult cottonwood, you may need to stop and take a few deep belly breaths to get the true feel of her/him.

Look and Learn: Cottonwoods are big enough and tall enough to be guideposts for the prairieland traveler. On the other hand, if you're hoping for a mountaintop or a virtual reality headset to be your guide, you may be looking in all the wrong places.

When you want to know more about who your granddaughter is dating now, you first look at his photo to see if he is cute enough for her. Then you read his bio to see if he really measures up. At least that's what Grandma Sue does, and I think it's all good effort that should also apply to nature's wonders.

If you really want to know cottonwood, a trip to the library (or an internet visit) can add to your understanding. For example, I didn't know there are male and female cottonwoods until an internet article on cottonwoods told me so. Nor did I know that the Biblical Balm of Gilead was likely made from the sticky resin found in black cottonwood tree buds, but now I do.

Traditional people – because they could sense that the cottonwoods around them connected their world to both the underworld and to the skies above – considered the trees to be spiritual Beings. Then, as messengers from above, the cottonwoods became symbols of hope, healing, and transformation (or regeneration).

Listen: Cottonwoods are perhaps the easiest of all the plants to listen to – their leaves quite literally speak with the urgings of the lightest of breezes. But some plant scientists and additionally some "attuned plant folk" claim that the plants speak to one another, to other beings, and even to us … if we'd just learn how to listen.

Respect: Many American Indigenous peoples respect the cottonwoods and honor them for their ability to connect and to provide hope and healing. The Lakota, for example, select a cottonwood to be the centerpiece and focal point of annual Sun Dance ceremonies.

I think there are lots of ways we can show our respect for those beings in Nature. We can simply give a tip-o-the-hat as we walk by, or add a "how ya doin buddy?" or a "god bless," or a "what's up pardner?" or a "Ho Mitakuye Oyasin." Or you can become a "tree hugger" and you can learn if you are one of those who, while you are hugging, can sense the pulse of the tree as its sap works its way up and down the trunk. Or …well you get the idea.

To my way of thinking, a simple act of respect is the very best mind-cleanser the world has to offer.

III

Last Words: In my conversations with Cottonwood, I was having a hard time relating to their ability to provide hope and I wondered how their symbolism of regeneration applied to me.

I knew from the get-go, after all, that my cancer (contrary to what the oncologists might try to tell me) was terminal, and that providing false hope might be more detrimental than helpful for me. I also knew that my days of regenerating my species were long past. Hell's sake, my youngest was born almost six decades ago.

And so, I thought of Cottonwood as a just and righteous symbol for Others … but not for me.

But wait just a minute. Maybe I should stop and listen to cottonwood's deeper message. With my ears wide open, the message then becomes one of hope for the next generations I helped create (the re-generations): I can have hope for my kids, grandkids, and great grandkids. And perhaps I can still do something to help justify that hope.

Then too, even as my body parts become no longer functional, I just might be able – as the cottonwood does – to create some kind of space or opening in my façade where the next generations can find hope, healing, and transformation ... perhaps even solace and security.

And finally, there's the message about aging and dying – with grace and dignity. Perhaps listening to the wisdom of cottonwood can help me with that too.

And so it is.

Rabbits

I

Introduction: Spring has sprung, so it's that time of year once again. I've been seeing lots of rabbits on my walks lately, and just today, Sue and I spotted a couple of happy bunnies "Doin' the Binky" as we were sauntering along on one of our walking trails.

There's something about rabbits (in addition to their uplifting "binky dance") that is lifting to the spirits. Something about watching the hop-away of a bouncing white tail that asks the mind to reach into the depths of its ability to dream, begs for a quickening of its capacity to imagine. Something about that cuddly little fur ball that makes you want to squeeze it to your chest, to smooth the fur, perhaps to nuzzle one of those long ears.

All this, of course, supposes that you are *not* seeing that damned rabbit as he is munching on your prized garden vegetables. That's the other side to rabbits (and to many of our common backyard critters): They are cute enough … unless they're destroying one of our human creations.

And additionally, many of our backyard critters, including rabbits, are so commonly seen we tend to not see them at all – unless, of course, they are devouring our stuff.

II

Rabbits Personified: Most folks know that rabbits breed like, well, like rabbits. And they know that rabbits love the gardener's lettuce. But rabbits are far more interesting and mysterious than this, and they seem to have a spirit that matches their cuteness and apparent guile. For example:

Pet Rabbits: Keeping a domesticated variety of rabbit as a pet can capture some of the magic and spirit of those cottontails you see in the wild. There are about 50 breeds of domesticated rabbits, ranging in size from the wee furball, to a rabbit as big as a large dog. Some of these breeds are recommended for first-time rabbit-owners; others are decidedly not. What's more, while cuddly rabbits may look like they'd be an easy-to-care-for addition to the family, they all require special care.

Special care includes: Their digestive system is easily upset without proper nutrients, including plenty of fiber; they have nasty reproductive-system diseases and cancers, which means that both males and females need to be spayed or neutered; and, because their incisors continue to grow throughout their lifetime, they have an absolute need to chew on things – things like furniture and electric cords.

Finally, a pet rabbit can live for 20 years or more, and thus will require a long-time commitment to its care and keeping.

I think most folks know by now that they should leave any baby rabbits (kits) they find in the wild alone, even if it seems they've been abandoned by mommas, and there are several good reasons for this. For starters, a kit's stomach has a pH that's ideal for bacterial growth. Fortunately for the kits, their stomach contains a protective antimicrobial factor called "milk oil." Milk oil is produced when a doe's milk comes in contact with enzymes in the kit's digestive tract. Hand-raised rabbits lack this protective antimicrobial factor which makes them susceptible to infections.

Rabbits Talk: The first rabbit I heard "talking" happened in my holistic veterinary practice as I was doing acupuncture and chiropractic adjustments on pet rabbits ... without really knowing much about what I was doing. Thing is: a lot of my patients got better, and I can only attribute this to their innate ability to absorb the positive chi energetics of acupuncture and chiropractic.

I remember when one of my first rabbit acupuncture patients, after I'd put all the needles in, started what sounded like purring. I wasn't sure what I was hearing, and asked the rabbit's owner. "Yeah, doc," she said, "when you're doing something that feels good, they purr. Congratulations to you for making her feel better."

A rabbit's purr doesn't come from its throat as a cat's purr does; it comes from a light grinding of their teeth. But they also have other words to say:

They hum, sometimes just for the hell of it, but more commonly it's the sound of a buck wooing his lady love. They hiss to ward off other rabbits; and if they are really afraid, they foot stomp or foot thump (thus Thumper the Rabbit). They whine or whimper when they don't want to be handled, or a doe might whine when she is pregnant and a buck is making unwanted advances. The sound of teeth grinding (not just lightly rubbing their teeth together as with a purr, but really grinding) indicates they are in a lot of pain. And they can let out a scream that will send chills down your spine ... whenever a predator makes a grab for them.

Rabbit's Spirited Reproduction: The phrase "breeding like rabbits" is not mere metaphor. One female rabbit and her offspring can theoretically produce 50,653 rabbits in three years, 69 million in five years, and 64 BILLION in seven years. (Compare this to similar calculations for a single female cat that can produce 120,000 kittens in seven years – and one human who can produce, what, 5 or so little babies in seven years.) And yes, all these calculations assume that no offspring are lost to predators or other natural causes, which, of course, does not happen. Still, 64 billion is one hell of a horde of rabbits from one momma.

Female rabbits are induced ovulators, meaning that ovulation occurs after breeding, and fertilization thus can occur whenever she accepts the advances of a buck. Periods of receptivity last anywhere from 5 to 14 days and are followed by one to ten days when they are not receptive – female rabbits can have from one to seven litters in a year. Gestation is 30 days, and results in litter sizes of from one to twelve; baby "kits" are weaned in a little over a month. Overall, rabbits average three to four litters per year, with the average number of kits being five.

Wild rabbits can alter both litter size and frequency of breeding during a season, an ability called "reproductive plasticity." This ability to either increase or decrease the number of young rabbits relies mostly on the amount of forage available – lots of greens, and does can gear up with increased numbers of ovulated eggs and by shortening the period between litters. Less available greens, and litter sizes and the number of kits per litter decrease.

Rabbit's Unusual Eating Habits: Gardeners know that rabbits like to take a nibble here, another there ...until they've destroyed an entire crop of new lettuce. But there's another eating habit of rabbits that may surprise you: they eat their own fecal pellets which are also known as cecotropes or night pellets, and they typically eat them directly from the source.

But, being very fastidious eaters, they choose only certain fecal pellets: usually those in the early morning, those that are mucus enclosed. It's a rabbit's way, since they don't have the four stomachs of a ruminant animal, to aid digestion by reintroducing beneficial bacteria that have been fermenting in the cecum (a large pouch that's connected to the junction of the small and large intestines).

Rabbits at Play: Early mornings and evenings are play times, the time when bunnies romp and cavort – in rabbit parlance it's called a binky and the internet has several videos showing the rabbit binky. There's so much spirit involved – they run and leap, turn cartwheels and flips, kick and prance. It's a wonder, with all that spinning and jumping, they don't, as I would certainly do, throw their backs out.

III

Rabbits vs Hares: Although they look somewhat alike, rabbits and hares are completely different species, and there are several noticeable differences between them. Hares are larger than rabbits and have longer hind legs and ears. Rabbits make their homes in burrows underground (our cottontail is an exception to this), while hares (and cottontails) nest above ground. Baby rabbits (kits) are born hairless and blind; hare babies (leverets) are born with hair and sight, and they can move about on their own shortly after birth. Rabbits tend to prefer softer grasses for their diet; hares like to eat bark and twigs. The two species of Jackrabbit seen in Kansas, the Whitetail and the Blacktail, are both hares.

IV

Rabbit as Trickster: Most of us think of Coyote as being the trickster, but different cultures have different models for their tricksters: fox, crow or raven, bluejay, raccoon, bear, spider and others occur in Native American myth. Rabbit appears as the primary trickster figure in many cultures, and is especially prevalent in Japanese culture. The antics of tricksters are often held up as examples of actions that are considered to be immoral, objectionable, or otherwise offensive to the culture in general. Some cultures even parody the trickster actions by ceremonially ridiculing them – to further etch into the human consciousness the importance of cultural mores.

Our own culture and folklore literature has several rabbit-as-trickster examples, including: Brer Rabbit, Bugs Bunny, The Tortoise and the Hare, and more.

V

Rabbit in the Moon. With all the spirit and tricksterism circling around the rabbit, it's no wonder she has found her place on the moon. While our culture insists there's a man in the moon, many other cultures see a rabbit – often one who is using a mortar and pestle to grind medicines that she will then spill onto us humans below ... to sprinkle us with some spirit-of-rabbit essence.

VI

Last Words: My impression is that rabbits need a better PR agent; someone to improve their general status among us humans. Or, maybe if we'd just stop, look, learn, and listen ... maybe then we'd have more respect for them.

Chapter 30 Interlude:
Some Rabbit Terms

Binky: A rabbit binky is when they jump and twist, sometimes in both directions one after another, before landing. Bunny binkies are a common rabbit behavior that expresses their happiness and comfort. A half-binky is when the rabbit does a little head flick – which also expresses, in rabbit body language, extreme joy. I'm not sure what a half-binky with a Salchow followed by a single Lutz and then a double axel would look like.

Bunny: Early 17th century – originally used as a term of endearment to a person, later as a pet name for a rabbit

Cecotropes (also known as cecal pellets and night pellets): These are fecal pellets that rabbits ingest to reintroduce bacteria into their digestive system.

Fluffle: A group of bunnies

Lagomorphs: Members of the taxonomic order, Lagomorpha, of which there are two living families: the Leporidae (rabbits and hares) and the Ochotonidae (pikas)

Mad as a March Hare: An English phrase derived from the observed antics – boxing with each other, jumping and leaping for no apparent reason, and in general acting a fool – antics said to occur only during the March breeding season of the European hare. The phrase is now used to describe any other animal or human who behaves in the excitable and unpredictable manner of a March Hare.

Rabbit Hole (or rabbit-hole, or rabbithole): A complexly bizarre or difficult state or situation that is mentally deranging, or disorienting – a state often conceived of as a hole (or rabbit burrow) into which one falls or descends.

"Falling down a rabbit hole" is often applied to the pursuit of something (such as an answer or solution) that leads to other questions, problems or pursuits – the rabbit hole a metaphor for something that transports someone into a wonderfully (or troublingly) surreal state or situation.

The rabbit hole, as popularized in "Alice's Adventures in Wonderland," symbolizes a portal that opens into new worlds, adventures, and unknown territories. The new world may be, depending on the interpreter (and the mental state of the interpreter): a psychedelic experience, deep-dream state, or a shamanic journey.

Scut: A short erect tail as of a rabbit, hare, or deer – (and possibly, or so I've been told, the tail on Playboy bunnies – which were initially made of yarn, but by 1969, had to be replaced by fire-retardant fake fur because customers were always trying to light them. But I digress.) Also "scut work" – from medical argot meaning: routine and often menial labor, oftentimes the work required of residents.

Thumper's Rule (aka: Thumperian Principle or Thumper's Law): "If you can't say something nice, don't say nothing at all." From Thumper, the rabbit in Disney's 1942 animated film *Bambi*.

Warren: A network of wild rabbit burrows. Recently extended to include other animals, as in a prairie dog warren.

White Rabbit: Rabbits, especially those with white fur, are a symbol of longevity in traditional Chinese culture. The ancient Chinese believed that the white rabbit was an incarnation of Alioth, the brightest star of the Triones.

One theory has it that if you follow the white rabbit – as seen in the story Alice in Wonderland, it will ultimately lead you to the truth, whatever that may be; or in other words, chasing a white rabbit means to chase the impossible, a fantasy, a dream. In this story-line, the white rabbit symbolizes one's curiosities and the lengths people are willing to go to satiate them.

Jefferson Airplane's "White Rabbit" is a song that supposedly takes the listener down the same psychedelic road Alice in the novel Alice in Wonderland journeys down.

Year of the Rabbit: Rabbit is one of the 12 animal signs of the Chinese zodiac. The sign of rabbit is a symbol of longevity, peace, and prosperity. People born in Rabbit years are described as vigilant, witty, quick-minded, ingenious, kind, smart, and docile. The year 2023, starting from January 22nd, 2023 and ending on February 9th 2024, is a *Year of the Rabbit.*

Snakes

I

Introduction: Snakes offer us a huge panoramic vista of what it is like to be an integral part of nature. There is no other species that opens for us quite the yawning portal into Nature's subtleties and nuances.

Think of the extremes of the human psyche's passionate emotions ... and snakes incite all of them: love/hate; fear and loathing/sensuous sexuality; demonic forces below/godly spirits above; venom and death/healing and regeneration. No other creature is a signifier, symbol, embodiment ... of so many opposing forces of Nature.

II

Snakes In Real Time: Snakes as symbols, snakes as gods, snakes as companions of the gods, and snakes as human companions, sexual and otherwise, are all well and good; snakes actually seen and interacted with are another matter entirely.

Watching snakes in motion, once your heart rate gets back to normal, is akin to viewing any highly trained athlete in action. There is simply no movement in nature that matches the snake's ability to effortlessly go from being fully stretched out and at-ease, into a tightly coiled body with head raised, cocked and ready to strike out faster than the blink of an eye.

III

Real Snakes: I have met a few snakes in my day – the serpentine, scaley, close-to-earth kind. Some of them face to face. Most of the face-to-face encounters have been with harmless black rat snakes, a common Kansas variety.

Once, when the birds in our portable chicken coop were setting up a racket, I decided to take a look-see. When I lifted the
hatch that opened into the nesting and egg laying area, I was
eye-to-eye with the dirty little egg-sucking black rat snake that
had been causing all the ruckus – he who had coiled up and then
extended neck and head, with forked-tongue flickering to taste
who I was.

Another time I was in the barn, trying to dig a sparrow nest
out of the rafters with a pitchfork when … a black rat snake literally jumped out of the nest in the rafters, twisting in the air, flying straight toward my left ear lobe. I ducked, he missed, landed
on the gate I was standing on and slithered away, leaving me
with a very sore pair of family jewels, the result of over-reacting
to a snake while pulling a wedgie on a barn gate. If I'd just have
left him alone, he would have taken care of my sparrow problem
himself.

There have been encounters with poisonous snakes too,
mostly copperheads on our farmstead. One reared up and came
straight at Sue and me while we were blissfully taking our daily
walk, struck at my left leg once, twice, missed both times (thanks
to my knee-jerk), and was gone. Another encounter with a coiled
and ready-to-strike copperhead on another part of our trail end-
ed with me successfully calming her down with some Reiki energy … and with us – me, Pokey the dog, and copperhead – becoming lasting friends for years to come.

Other snakey encounters also evolved into long-term friend-
ships: The beautiful Red-sided Garter snake that helped keep
our garden free of vermin and that I would see scurrying away
whenever I mowed around the garden. The black rat snake that
kept trying to lay eggs in a pile of compost at the edge of our
yard – me hauling her, dangling at the end of a rake, back into
the woods time after time after time … until Sue finally took her
eggs into the woods, and momma snake quit coming back too.

Now that we live in the city, I actually miss the brief jolt of
adrenaline that comes with snake sightings … although I've seen
a few snakes even here. There was the cute little Ring-necked
snake I moved off the sidewalk of the apartment complex next
door, figuring he might cause a stir if he stayed there. And the
Prairie Rat snake – he who looks a lot like a copperhead (to me

at least). And the huge Black Rat snake that Sue spotted, just lying there next to a rock outcropping alongside the sidewalk that runs along Wakarusa Street (one of Lawrence's major arteries), sunning, likely just emerged from her hibernaculum.[25]

Unfortunately, most of the snakes I see here in the city are now flattened fauna. For me: one of the shames of city life; for the snakes: one of the hazards of city life.

IV

Snakes In the Environment: Living, breathing snakes are actually a vital part of the ecology of any natural environment.

To begin with, they are predators, and their usual prey – small rodents such as rats, mice, moles, voles – are the carriers of a host of diseases, including: Plague, Salmonellosis, Tularemia, Leptospirosis, Hantavirus, and Rat-Bite Fever. These same rodents are secondary carriers (via the ticks and fleas they are infested with) of diseases such as: Rocky Mountain Spotted Fever, Murine Typhus, Lyme Disease and West Nile Virus. Could we say that Snake has earned her place on the staff of Asclepius?

Acting as predators, snakes offer several other benefits: those little rodents they consume are seed eaters, with bellies and cheek pouches full of seeds – seeds that find their way through the snake's gut undigested and end up being planted. Snake plantings roam far and wide – their home range is much wider than the rodents who supplied them with the seeds. Could we say that Snake is the Johnny Appleseed of the lower world?[26]

Because they eat little rodents and thus ingest and bioaccumulate all the stuff the rodents have been exposed to, snakes have been used to monitor the area's levels of organic pollutants: pesticides, polychlorinated biphenyls, dioxin-related compounds, plasticizers, etc. Snakes have even been used to monitor the radiation levels of fallout at sites such as Fukushima. Could

---

25 A hibernaculum is a protected place where various creatures spend the winter in order to avoid the cold weather. Examples include: insects, bats, snakes, and some mammals. A lone animal (such as a bear) might seek a hibernaculum, or several hundred animals (including many snake species) may congregate together.

26 The black rat snake we saw sprawled out in the weeds apparently decided it was too early to leave the hibernaculum – she made a tight 180° turn and slowly climbed back up the layers of exposed limestone and shale, found the tiny opening into the rocks she had crawled out of, and disappeared.

we say that Snake has replaced the canary-in-the-mineshaft?

Yes, snakes also eat birds and bird eggs too, and cutesy little bunnies, and baby critters of all ilk, and even the occasional wee pet dog or cat (especially in Florida where the escaped pet pythons and boas have taken over the swamplands).

V

Snake Imagery: There's more to snakes than fear and loathing; they also offer unique opportunities for imagery, both good and bad. A few examples follow:

Ouroboros: One of the earliest of the snake symbolisms is a zero – or perhaps better thought of as the Big O. The ouroboros is the emblematic serpent of ancient Egypt and Greece, represented as a large snake (or dragon) in a circle with its tail in its mouth, continually devouring its own body and then being reborn from itself. Or, the O of the ouroboros may be twisted in its middle, becoming what we now know as the symbol for infinity.

The story of the German chemist, Kekulé, takes the ouroboros to a new level: The story goes that Kekulé's head was spinning, trying to determine the chemical structure of the organic gas, benzene … when it hit him during a dream. Benzene, in the dream, became an ouroboros representing a spinning hexagonal ring of six carbon atoms twisting and turning like a snake. Organic chemistry's origins thus wedded to ouroboros.

Life Force: Historically, serpents and snakes have represented fertility or a creative life force. As snakes shed their skin through sloughing to reveal a slick, brand-new outer coat, they are symbols of rebirth, transformation, immortality, and healing.

Healing professions typically incorporate the image of two snakes in the Caduceus: The original Greco/Roman god of medicine was Asclepius, son of Apollo. The healing rod that Asclepius carried with him, depending on the storyteller, might represent the traveling physician of the day, walking along with the help of his cane … or the cane could represent the human spine. The wrapped-around snake (Asclepius's cane had only one snake wrapped around it) might be symbolic of both the regenerative healing and the potentially poisonous effects of snakes ... or it might simply have been "medicine" to ward off the effects of a poisonous snake bite. (Asclepius is said to have learned how to avoid death after watching snakes use herbs to treat themselves.)

As a different symbol entirely, two snakes wrapped around a rod with attached wings were traditionally associated with Hermes and Mercury – gods of commerce and negotiation. When this symbol is used by entities of BigPharma and BigMed and ReallyBigOncoMed, the irony of the two-faces of snakes becomes evermore apparent.

Gods: In addition to being related to healing and medicine, images of snakes have crawled their way into the pantheon of gods in almost all cultures. Several images of snake gods have been recovered from Sumerian Mesopotamia, and the ancient Egyptians worshiped snakes, especially the cobra, believing that the cobra was associated with the sun god Ra.

More God Snakes: In ancient Greece there was the serpent god, Ophion; in Italy, the serpent goddess, Marisan, who is associated with witches, snakes, snake-charmers … and healing. In Hindu the god Shiva is often depicted with a cobra coiled around his neck, and the Indian cobra, *Naja naja*, symbolizes his mastery over the world-illusion. Vishnu, another of the Hindu gods, is usually portrayed as reclining on the coiled body of a giant snake deity with multiple cobra heads.

Before his enlightenment, Buddha (Siddhartha), is often shown seated on the coils of a giant naga (snake or serpent) as he meditated. While sitting there, so the story goes, he was shielded from a raging storm by a huge cobra … so he could continue his meditation and achieve eventual salvation.

And lest we forget, in Genesis 3:1 there is the prominent appearance of a snake in the Garden of Eden – a snake presence of many differing interpretations. Was the serpent the devil or Satan incarnate – or merely a trickster entity, a representation of cunning and evil? Only the shadow of the apple tree knows.

And, so it goes – snakes have been worshiped either as gods or as signifiers of regeneration and reproduction, wisdom and cunning, healing and medicine.

VI

Last Words: Love em or hate em; worship them or fear them – snakes are a part of our environment … even here in the city.

Chapter 31 Interlude:
Fear (and Love) of Snakes

I

Fear of Snakes: Fear of snakes is likely an inherited trait in almost every world culture, and the fear seems to be hard-wired – even human toddlers and the babies of some monkey species react to snakes (or photos of snakes) … or they quickly learn to react. This fear seems likely to have evolved as protection from potentially harmful snakes – even in countries such as ours, where snakes are not a real problem. CDC estimates that 7,000 to 8,000 people are bitten annually by venomous snakes in the United States … but only about five of those bitten die.

And yes, some 10 to 40 percent of those bitten by rattlesnakes end up with lasting injuries such as losing the function of or a part of a finger. But, you actually have a better chance of dying from lightning strike than from snakebite. Around 400 to 500 people in the U.S. are struck by lightning each year; about 10% of the strikes are lethal – by my reckoning, about 40 to 50 deaths per annum, or about 10 times the deaths caused by snake bite. Lightning strikes that don't kill, do often leave the surviving 90% with varying forms of disability … and hopefully the good sense to come in out of the rain the next time.

Worldwide, of course, venomous snakes are a more real problem. WHO estimates that about 5.4 million people worldwide are bitten each year, causing death in 80,000 to 138,000 of those bitten, and around three times as many amputations and other permanent disabilities are caused by snake bites annually. We get off easier because the U.S. has better healthcare and more rapid access to it.

To ponder: As climate change brings us more heat, more and

more of those tropics-loving venomous snakes will be traveling northward, slithering up our way.

Ophidiophobia: The mere sight of a snake in the grass (even if it's a picture of a snake in the grass) will cause a degree of anxiety in roughly 50% of all people. What's more, 2 to 3 percent of the population has ophidiophobia, an extreme fear of snakes that, upon confronting a snake, can produce severe and often debilitating physical reactions that might include: sweating, nausea, increased heart and/or breathing rates, dizziness, hot flashes or chills, tremors, burning or prickly feelings in your extremities, and diarrhea ... along with audible screaming.

II

Snake Love: And finally, on the other side of the coin, love for snakes (*ophidiophilia*) seemingly knows no bounds. Some folks have a sex kink that involves animals, and one sub-type of that fetish is *ophidicism*, defined as a woman (usually, or occasionally a man) whose sexual arousal hinges on the use of a reptile's tail as a sex object (usually it's the tail, although occasionally heads are also used). I have not been an eyewitness to such antics, so I'll leave it to your own imagination to figure out just how this works.

III

Last Words: Ah, the nuances and extremes represented by nature ... some of which I have no words to describe.

Nutty Squirrels

I

Introduction: It is my first autumn, post-cancer diagnosis, and I am walking as if I own the sidewalks now – upright with walking sticks … and I think rather jauntily. The squirrels are not in agreement with my assessment. They chirp at me from the back side of the trees, warning me to stay the hell on my side of the walkways and to quit bothering them while they are working.

Their oaks are turning from green to brilliant reds and brownish-reds, and *their* acorns are ripe for the harvest.

The squirrels are a hoot to watch as they skitter about, working to supply the larder for the winter months ahead. You better believe that they own the trees they scamper around on, and woe betide anyone who tries to tell them any different. They announce their ownership as they hang, often upside down from the side of the tree just out of view – their ever-active nose and beady eyes barely visible from just under a hideaway limb. But, their chatterings are as clear as the sound of nuts cracking.

II

Nutty Squirrels: Someone who is "squirrely" is seen as someone who is restless, nervous, fidgety, eccentric – and that surely describes squirrels for most of the year, but especially in the fall when nuts, their favorite food, are ripe.

Fall is the time of year when tree squirrels nervously fidget from nut to nut, restlessly selecting the best of the fallen crop, which they then bury, each prized nut deposited in a separate *cache* (or *midden*). A bit eccentric maybe, but the method gives them a supply of nuts to last over the winter months – actually a decent, rational strategy, since they don't hibernate and thus need a food supply throughout the winter.

Watch closely and you'll note that the hoarders select a nut, handle each one, shake it and flick their head, and perhaps put it into their mouth for a brief taste. Then, they'll turn the nut over several times in their paws (known as *paw manipulation*). All this is to test whether that nut meets their needs or not. A nut that rattles might indicate the presence of a weevil inside, and that nut will likely be eaten right away, weevil and all. Other nuts are sorted by size, feel and smell ... and then stored in individual holes that are arranged in a manner easy to remember.

A single gray or fox squirrel can stash hundreds or even thousands of individual caches in a year. The most logical reason for a squirrel to hoard its nuts in a scattering of spots is that it makes it more difficult for another animal – say, another squirrel, a chipmunk, or raccoon – to steal the winter's supply in one fell swoop.

The caching squirrel will use several methods of subterfuge when burying his nuts – including digging several ghost holes that don't contain any nuts and fake burying of one nut in several places.

But biologists have discovered several other aspects to scatter hoarding that make the squirrel even more eccentric than originally thought.

III

Cognition and Brain Power: The head flick, coupled with paw manipulation, gives the squirrel a wealth of information about the nut: its weight, how fresh it is, if it is insect-infested, is the shell intact, and how best to transport it to its hiding place. Bigger nuts, like walnuts, are buried at a lower density than smaller nuts, like acorns – a strategy that keeps marauders from discovering a rich stash.

But the squirrels are also smart enough to use *"spatial categorization"* (also known as *"spatial chunking"*) when burying their nuts – a method that puts walnuts in one area and acorns and hickory nuts in another. Testing of humans and lab animals has shown that it is easier to remember where things are if you've got them organized. And so it is that the squirrels build a mental map of their nut caches. (All this assumes that, unlike someone my age, they can remember what it is they have come into the room to get in the first place.)

But does this spatial categorization actually work? Various studies show that squirrels recover from 40 to 80% of the nuts they have buried. While this may seem like a wide gap in nuts recovered, there is at least one reason for the discrepancy: some squirrels are just smarter than others. Well, duh.

Questions remain: Do they actually remember where they stored all those nuts? Or do they smell the nuts in the ground? Or do they randomly dig until they find a nut? Most researchers think they probably use some sniffing to find their cache, but squirrels also seem to be as accurate at finding nuts during snow cover when odors wouldn't travel through the snow – pointing to at least some memory involvement.

Watch a squirrel scoring a nut in winter, and you'll see a nimble scamper down the tree, a scurry to the cache site, and a furious dig and rapid return to the tree. Eluding predators and thus survival depends on quickness; there's not enough time to sniff under every fallen oak leaf. This quick-as-a-squirrel activity further supports the effects memory has on the ability to recover nuts.

There's another key to squirrel intelligence: **brain growth**. As they are hunting for and caching a long winter's supply of nuts, their brains actually grow bigger. During the fall ripe-nut season, a squirrel's brain is larger than at any other time of the year.[27] Off-season it recedes back to a smaller size.

IV

Our Squirrely Ancestors: According to most (but not all) paleontologists, the world's oldest and most primitive mammal was *Purgatorius*, a tiny squirrel-like creature that spent much of its time climbing trees and eating fruits and nuts. Beginning some 60-odd million years ago, good old *Purgatorius* was hanging from his hind legs, much like the squirrels of today do. And for the 10 million-or-so years he acted as our most primitive ancestor, he was probably chirping at passers-by.

---

27 Specifically, the hippocampus, which is the memory and spatial organization area of the brain, increases 15% in size in the fall.

The hang-by-their-back-legs ability of squirrels (and *Purgatorius*) is a result of their ankle anatomy which allows it to turn a full 180^0. Comparatively, as we humans developed the ability to stand upright, we dropped our heel down so we could walk on a flattened-out accumulation of metatarsal bones, rather than on the little phalanges (toes). The human heel bone (which in other mammals is the hock) became locked in a rear-pointing position, and we humans could no longer turn our feet 180^0.

Had we kept our squirrely ankles, we could have rotated our feet front to back … and would thus have had a logical reason for not knowing whether we were coming or going. We would also likely have been able to jump a lot higher than we can today … thus maybe allowing me to, at long last, dunk a basketball. Or jump from one tree to another. Ah, progress … and its limitations.

But wait! There's more – another body oddity of the squirrel: the size of his testicles ebbs and flows, according to the breeding seasons. During breeding seasons (typically late winter and again in mid summer) the squirrel's testicles can grow to huge proportions. (For the curious: there are internet images aplenty of the squirrel's huge family jewels.)

Then, when the breeding season has come and gone, the testicles (and the prostate) recede in size. When the testicles are fully reduced in size, they recede back into the abdominal cavity – which has led to the folklore that squirrels, for whatever nutty reason, chew each other's nuts off. So much for fake news folklore.

V

Last Words: Seems that evolution can take some odd-ball twists and turns … for better or for worse.

Chapter 32 Interlude:
Squirrels and Cancer

Introduction: Turns out that our nutty squirrels (and their cousins, naked mole rats, chipmunks, muskrats, and chinchillas) may have a few stories to tell us about how to avoid cancer. So, to set the stage:

There are two biochemicals found in most cells that are integral to the development of most cancers: telomeres and telomerase. Like most things in nature their involvement is a complex web of interactions – good and bad – and so far, much of the untangling of the intricate web has been done in laboratory flasks. But our squirrely rodents may have the key to unlocking a way for us to avoid cancers.

Telomeres are the caps at the end of each strand of cellular DNA that protect our chromosomes, much like the plastic tips at the end of shoelaces. Without these caps, the DNA strands in our cells become damaged, much like shoelaces without tips become frayed. As our cells divide, the end segment of the telomere is lopped off, and when a telomere is shortened beyond a certain limit, the cell no longer divides … thus old age ensues and eventually death.

Another result of a frayed chromosomal end is that the cells can get befuddled and confused, and the altered cell then has a greater chance to mutate into a cancer cell. When this happens, all the king's horses and all the king's men won't be able to put the "Humpty Dumpty" cell back together again.

Telomerase is an enzyme that helps telomeres maintain their length, which, in turn, helps the cells maintain their ability to divide and thus stay alive. Telomerase is found in rapidly dividing cells such as sperm and epithelial cells, but it is usually absent in other slowly-dividing bodily (somatic) cells. Some scientists believe that telomerase is the key to aging slowly and thus to long life.

On the other hand, telomerase is active in about 90% of the various types of cancer cells. In tumors, telomerase acts as the enzyme that allows the cancer cells to grow to abnormal size and numbers. So: to enhance telomerase activity; or not to enhance. Damned if you do; damned if you don't.

II

Squirrels, Cancer, and Telomerase: Squirrels and their cousins are relatively long-lived – the common grey squirrel may live 24 years or more. And, over all that time they have very active telomerase ... which should make them susceptible to high rates of cancer. However, squirrels rarely (if ever) get cancer. It appears that squirrels have evolved another mechanism for using telomerase to their advantage ... while at the same time, curtailing its ability to cause cancer.

So what gives? Well, the answer isn't yet clear – Nature doesn't disclose Her secrets easily. But there is hope at the end of the tunnel. Hope that this time we will use the holistic aspects of Nature to give us the answers ... instead of using the war metaphor as our model while we search for a silver bullet to blast away at the invading cancer cells.

Ecological Answers: Squirrels (and many other animals and plants) use what is called reproductive plasticity to alter their rate of reproduction – when times are good, reproduction rates increase; bad times reduce rates. There are many factors involved, including whether food supplies are up or down, and whether predators are rare or abundant.

But, here again, it seems to me that perhaps a holistic ecological approach to evaluating the why behind how cancer decides to increase cell reproductive rates and cellular size might offer more valid answers, better solutions ... rather than continuing to think that going to war against the rogue cells is the only way to deal with cancer.

Up and Down Cell Growth: This is just me thinking again, but couldn't the answer lie in the emotions, perhaps along with biochemical and eco-systemic solutions? Remember that the squirrel grows and then shrinks both brain cells and testicular (and prostatic) cells during specific times of the seasons. And these seasonal changes occur during periods of intense emotional joy: the seasons of lust and of being able to dine on one's favorite foods.

And so, wouldn't it be just peachy keen if the final answer to Nature's Rubix Cube of cancer would be to find and enhance our joy – which would then let our cells grow in response… only to recede until we needed another hit of joy juice.

As I say, just thinkin' here.

III

Last Words: Well, to my way of thinking, there may be hope for us as a species after all. Light and hope at the end of the tunnel. Hope that doesn't involve a war metaphor requiring a scorched earth protocol that ends up blowing us up … along with the tunnel.

Cedar

I

Introduction: I've recently discovered a gravel-covered walking trail that begins at the new police station and winds its way through woodsy cover that is mostly Eastern Red Cedar. On my early morning walks the air is alive with the scent of cedar – it's a bit of a nose-prickling aroma, a fresh-air blast that awakens the senses, breathes positive energetics into the spirit, and adds an aha to the soul.

The Eastern Red Cedar, *Juniperus Virginiana*, is, as the name implies, actually a juniper, a slow-growing evergreen tree of the cypress family. It is a dioecious tree – pollen and seed cones are on separate trees. In September female trees produce the small, waxy purple balls that contain the seeds.

II

Cedars Yea and Nay: Not everyone in Kansas appreciates our cedars as much as I do. In fact, most folks hereabouts, especially ranchers, see the cedar tree as their mortal enemy.

The Red Cedar is native to Kansas, but it is considered a pioneer invader – which means that it is one of the first trees to repopulate cleared, eroded, or otherwise damaged land. It also means that, without proper control measures, it can become invasive. When it invades, a field of cedars soon becomes a mire of sticky, prickly needles that takes over the pasture, killing out undergrowth grasses and oftentimes becoming so dense that animals (like cattle) can't force their way through the interwoven limbs.

Around here you can tell it's springtime when you see clouds of smoke rising from the pasture fires. It's an annual ritual of renewal: burning off the dead grasses and the upstart cedars. If you had let those cedars grow for 10 years or so, you would have that impenetrable evergreen forest that can only be returned to usable pasture with the help of the bulldozer's blade.

Ranchers tell the story of newly-built paved roads being their biggest bugaboo: Roads bring more human pioneer invaders into the prairie (invaders that will then become settlers), and along with the human invasion comes the cedars … cedars that can't be burned because there are too many people around.

On the other hand, city folks tell their story of how the smoky pollution from the springtime prairie fires stifle the air from nearby to as far away as Omaha and beyond. (Omaha is roughly 300 miles northeast of the Flint Hills, the area in Kansas where most of the prairie burning occurs.)

There are still other folks, typically non-ranchers, who enjoy the fresh feel of a cedar woods, who appreciate the cedar for its ability to offer home-sites and hide-away areas for many bird and wild animal species, for the cedar tree's worth as a wild edible and medicinal herbal, for its elegant way of entering our folklore, and for the spiritual qualities it has provided for many cultures, including Native American cultures.

III

The Cedar Tree: The cedar's evergreen foliage provides nesting and roosting cover for several bird species, including sparrows, robins, mockingbirds, juncos, and warblers. Twigs and greenery are eaten by hooved browsers including deer, and the purple fruits are consumed by many animals, most extensively by cedar waxwings.

We had a huge cedar tree at the corner of our deck out on the farm, and every fall it attracted cedar waxwings by the dozens to feast on the berries. About two or three days and they had eaten their fill … and were gone for another year. Grandpa Shaw called them "cockatoos," and he kept track of their comings and goings by telling us that, "them cockatoos were here again last week, Monday I think it was."

Traditionally, a tea made from the leaves or berries has been used as a general tonic or to treat a variety of ailments, such as: canker sores, coughing, diarrhea, vomiting and bleeding. Young leafy twigs of the red cedar were officially listed in the U.S. Pharmacopoeia from 1820-1894, as a diuretic.

In my veterinary practice I made extensive use of the homeopathic remedy, *Thuja* – for treating warts, for mitigating the adverse side effects of medications, and for a variety of other conditions. Homeopathic Thuja is a remedy made from the *Thuja Occidentalis* tree -- aka: Eastern Arborvitae or Northern White Cedar, a close cousin to the Eastern Red Cedar.

Cedar berries are used to add flavor to soups, meats, and drinks (gin). To my way of thinking, however, the taste of cedar – whether as a flavoring or as a drink – is, um, not my cup of tea – too much bite; not enough sweet.

Eastern Red Cedars have the potential to live over 850 years (one in Missouri was estimated to be 705 years old); a normal red cedar will grow to a height of 40 to 50 feet, with much taller specimens not uncommon – growth rates are very slow, typically 1 to 1 1/2 feet per year.

After a youth of being year-round green and vibrant, greeting each day with outstretched arms; then after becoming teenager-trees, gathering together in tight-knit crowds and listening to the strum and thrum of the birds and bees while dancing to the winds; and finally, after anointing themselves in pungent aromas that everyone within miles can smell … our maturing cedars become more sedate, almost introverted, and they often go unnoticed, hiding behind other trees as they age and grow into craggy, shaggy, statuesque and wise old entities. Aged cedars have become Old-Man trees that seem to moan into the night air, complaining about the pains in their creaky limb-joints.

With a true-life story such as the cedar's, it is easy to see how they have become the subject of so many folktales, the authors of their own claim to spirituality.

Native Americans have traditionally used cedar as an incense and purifying herb. Cedar is commonly used in sweat lodge ceremonies, and many tribal members carry a small piece of cedar wood in their medicine bags, or they will place a piece above the household entrance for protection. Cherokee beliefs say that the cedar holds the spirits of the departed.

IV

Last Words: The cedar is known variably as the "tree of life" or the "graveyard tree," and it is a tree often seen growing in graveyards. It also seems that every region of our country has a folktale to tell about cedars and graveyards, or cedars and deaths, or cedars and spirits – both living and dead.

My favorite tale is an old Ozarks superstition that says: When the cedar tree you planted around your grave site grows tall enough to shade it, that's when you are due to die. Thankfully, cedars are slow growers; you wouldn't want the story to be about a fast-growing cottonwood.

And again thankfully, I am good with the thinking that my planted cedar may have grown tall enough to shade my gravesite. Thankful that I've lived my life to the best I could. Thankful that I'll have the shade of a cedar to comfort me … forever more.

Chapter 33 Interlude: Cedar

I

Cedar Afterwords: Just thinking here, but don't many of the negative-sided stories of cedar remind you of our own story – a story, after all, of a species of pioneer invader (us) becoming, often via massive migrations, invasive (the Oregon/ California Trails, as but one example here).

Could we not be considered an invasive species that has often rendered the land almost uninhabitable to those multiple *other* species that had previously roamed its open spaces? Us: an invasive species that has sucked the life out of soil and water and air … leaving our own fetid odors behind.

And in another vein entirely: Couldn't we visualize cancer cells as simply pioneer invaders that, left unchecked, might become invasive (metastatic) … demolishing and then eating all living cells in their way? And would it be possible, even slightly possible, to view cancer thusly – as a native species, becoming a pioneer invader that, without some controlling force, becomes invasive … leaving the footprints of invasion in the ruble left behind.

Buying into that bit of reasoning, the real question would be: if cancer cells could be viewed as Good-Old-Boy pioneers gone rogue – instead of treating them as invading armies that are intent, from the outset, on wreaking havoc and mayhem onto all things in their way … would that change the way we treat cancers?

Could we change the very basic ways we think about and treat cancer – by simply changing the cancer metaphor from being an act of cellular warfare into it being the movement of pioneer cells just out there looking for a better life?

Ahh, the forever changing landscape that Nature has to work with – with all of us mere players on Her stage. Ahh, the ongoing nuance of Nature; ahh the yin-yang of everything. Both nuance and yin-yang, always integral and vital parts of the storyline – a wide breadth of storyline tunneled into one person's visions … always with a light at the end of the tunnel.

As I say: Just thinking here.

PART FIVE: Death and Dying

How Long Has He Got Left

I

Introduction: It is August, 2019, and we have moved (*FINAL-LY!!*) into our new digs: the Village Cooperative of Lawrence (now renamed: Branchwood Village Senior Living Cooperative). One of the final tasks of moving is to change your address with all the folks that matter, and since we don't want the flow of money from the government to stop, Sue heads down to the Social Security Office to complete the paperwork. I'm still wobbly from the cancer surgery, and we figure that if we have all the documents in order and we live together, she can register for me. Apparently not so.

Sue: "Thanks for getting my paperwork finished. Now I need to get Randy's completed. He's my husband."

Government Guy: "He's got to come in personally."

Sue: But I have all his paperwork here: Birth certificate, driver's license, past year's tax returns, our new address, and…

Gov. Guy: "He's got to come in."

Sue: "But it's all here. Just like mine, and mine was OK."

Gov. Guy: He's got to come in."

So in exasperation, Sue pulls the cancer card, the ace in the hole that has already worked for us on many occasions: "Randy's got terminal cancer, and it's really tough for him to get around."

Gov. Guy, without changing expressions: "Well, how long has he got left? Because if it's not very long, he might not need to change his address anyway. The government is pretty slow getting paperwork done."

And so, Sue makes another appointment, and a few weeks later I wobble my way into the Social Security Office, paperwork in hand. But, the question lingers in my mind: "How long *has* he got left?"

II

Life Expectancy: It's not the first time I've confronted that question. I was asked to give a talk to our 55th high school reunion, class of 1960. As a part of the talk, I wanted to give us all something to brag about, something to be thankful for – something like the fact that, since we all had been born around 1942 (which made us all about 73 years old at the time), we had already outlived our life expectancy that, at the time of our birth, had been 68 years.

Already 5 years to the good … and I'm wondering: If I would spend my time more gracefully and be less bungling, how much longer *could* I have. This is, of course, before being diagnosed with cancer.

"Normal" Life Expectancy refers to the average number of years an individual, or a group of people, or a specific population is expected to live. Predicting life expectancy is, of course, not as easy as pulling a number out of a hat. It can be affected by a person's family and health history, genetics, income, level of education, living environment, lifestyle factors such as diet, and even race, age and sex. Females tend to live longer than males – something like 5 years longer.

Every year's birth population has a life expectancy, and until just recently that expectancy in the U.S. has risen every year. For example, the life expectancy of a person born in 2017 is 78.6 years – 76.1 years for male babies; 81.1 years for females. (This compares to the 68 years for those of us born in 1942.)

Other factors affect an individual's life expectancy. For example, many of life's more serious ailments occur in a person's earlier years. Thus, each year a person lives, they have survived multiple potential causes of death … which means that life expectancy actually can increase with age.

For instance: My life expectancy at birth – or that of any one of my classmates born in 1942 – was about 68 years. However, any one of us who had survived to age 65 could expect to live another 18.4 years – or to 83.4 years of age. If that person lived to 75, their life expectancy increased to 86.8 years, which is, interestingly, 9.3 years longer than what the average child born in 2006 has. When Sue and I hit our 78th birthday this September (we were born on the same day), she will have a life expectancy of 10.11 more years; a healthy me (that is, me without cancer) could expect to live 8.27 more years.

On the internet there are dozens of charts and graphs that provide various methods for determining one's life expectancy. Some are even interactive: you can plug in variables such as: whether or not you smoke; your occupation (some occupations are more dangerous than others); your diet; known diseases you have now or have had in the past; on and on. Why, I'd guess you could spend whatever time you have left looking at life expectancy charts and playing with their variables.

III

Cancer and Life Expectancy: There's a metaphor often used to describe how cancers work: the turtle, the rabbit, and the bird. Cancers tend to have characteristic rates-of-growth that mimic the typical speed of these three critters: a *turtle* slowly lumbers onwards; *rabbits* hippity hop along, then dash into the bushes, where they amble from one tasty bush to the next one, taking a nibble from each bush along the way; *birds*, once they've decided on their prey, can reach incredible speeds. Perhaps the fastest of any animal is the peregrine; a falcon that, under ideal conditions, can reach speeds of up to 200 mph{320 km/h}in a dive.

Turtle cancers creep along, and some of them progress so slowly that the patient will die of old age before the cancer can get them. At the other extreme, *bird cancers* at full-out speed and can fly along so fast it's almost impossible to find any cure that will stop them.

Finally, in between these two types of cancers are the *rabbit cancers,* the hop-along-at-varying-speeds cancers. These are the cancers that typically respond the best to a variety of therapies – treatments that can catch a rabbit in mid-hop or while nibbling … and can slow it down or even prevent it from moving along at all.

The creep-along characteristic of turtle cancers has created its own list of problems. Generally speaking, the earlier you catch a cancer, the easier it is to cure it. Thus, lots of effort has been given to devising tests to detect the cancer and ways of ensuring that large numbers of people get tested. But this methodology is not always the best for all people. Some people, for example, tend to overreact when they learn their test has come back positive, and these folks might be scared into thinking that they need procedures – such as surgeries, biopsies, or chemotherapies – that they really don't need.

With all cancers it's important to weigh the benefits of a particular therapy versus its "costs" – the likelihood and potential severity of adverse side effects. But with turtle cancers you should also weigh the probability that it might progress so slowly that old age will get you before the cancer does. Since all cancer treatments carry with them a certain amount of risk as well as "costs," the decision to treat a turtle cancer is not always an easy one.

A good example of turtle vs rabbit cancers: if you're an old guy – say over the age of 65 or 70 – when you are diagnosed with a typical turtle cancer (for example, prostate cancer Stage 1 or 2), you will likely die of old age before the cancer gets you. Prostate cancer Stage 4 is considered a rabbit cancer, with a normal life expectancy of about 3 to 5 years after diagnosis.

So, now that I have been diagnosed (at age 76) with a rabbit cancer (Stage 4 prostate cancer), I know that the rabbit will eventually hop and nibble its way to a meet-up with the guy with a scythe … no matter the therapy my oncologist and I choose to use.

IV

Me and My Oncology Doc: I, like so many other people with cancer, will be required to play the numbers game of lab results and of percentages … and how both of those relate to my expected years of longevity. My understanding of my New-World-With-Cancer depends on how well I can comprehend the garble of statistical probabilities, lab results, and blatant bullshit put out by the institution of BigOncologyMed. This is the burden every cancer patient must endure -- while they are also just hoping for a decent or even tolerable quality of life (QoL) … as they are also just trying to survive.

My Doc puts me on a chemotherapy regime whose aim is to kill the cancer cells that have spread to bones and other body parts throughout my body. But prostate cancer cells are conniving little bastards, and they will eventually find ways to regenerate and go about their merry way of body damage. You can slow down their march for a while with feminizing hormones, but even these treatments eventually lose their effectiveness.

After chemotherapy and just before beginning hormone treatments, I ask my Onc Doc, "How long have I got left?"

Doc: "Typically the hormones work for 20 to 22 months."

Me: "What then?"

Doc: "It will take one to three years for the cancer to grow back. So, unless we change to another type of therapy, you'll likely need to go into hospice somewhere within that one to three year time frame."

Me: "How do we tell when the hormones have stopped working?"

Doc: "We have your PSA (Prostatic Specific Antigen) levels down close to zero now, but they will ultimately begin to elevate again. When your PSA reaches 4.0, we know the hormones are no longer working. That's when it's time to change treatments."

My PSA initially was somewhere around 5,000 – the highest my Doc had ever seen. (Guess that makes me a one-percenter – Hi Ho, Hi Ho!) My last PSA, at my exam three months ago, had gone from 0.13 to 0.25. Expectations now are for it to have climbed to 4 or more.

I am now at 22 months into hormone treatment (the time predicted for when I would need to switch treatments), and I have just received perhaps my last hormone therapy. I have decided – for a number of reasons – that I will not opt for further therapy.

The reasons include: 1) Financial: available treatments at this time cost thousands of dollars per month; 2) Poor cost/benefit ratio: today's treatment options provide only a few months of increased longevity; and 3) Quality of Life: the incredible load of painful and debilitating side effects – physical, mental and emotional – that have come with this current hormone therapy have been such that I don't want to tolerate them any longer.

V

Possibilities: But wait: there is, according to my Doc, some new light at the end of the tunnel. Early work with a combination of two new cancer drugs has shown encouraging results. The next step for these drugs is to try them out on a number of patients – do a trial to see how they really work for lots of people.

According to my Doc, early results from short-term trials have shown promise – fewer adverse side effects, and some patients feel much better. Long term results are not yet available.

However, according to my reading of CDC's information about trial results so far: Adverse side effects have been about the same as with previous drugs in both number of patients affected and severity of effects. A few patients have reported feeling better than when on previous meds, but with every statistical model there's a tale of a very small number of respondents on the plus side of things – in the case of cancer treatments, of patients that live longer and have a better quality of life.

There is the fact that, being in the trial, I'd get the meds for free. Countered by the fact that it's a placebo-based trial, meaning I have a 50:50 (flip of the coin) chance to be one of the "lucky ones" getting the meds.

VI

What Are the Odds: But wait: we are now in the middle of the COVID-19 pandemic which has thrown a monkey wrench into all calculations of life expectancies.

First: Early experience indicates that certain populations – the elderly, people with current health problems (such as diabetes and obesity), those with cancer, and people of color – all have an increased likelihood of contracting the Covid virus and of dying from the infection.

Second: Covid infection rates will depend greatly on how people respond to the pandemic – whether or not people practice social distancing and wearing masks will be important factors.

Third: The ability to decrease death rates will ultimately depend on reliable and effective testing, subsequent isolation of reactors, and on how quickly **safe** and **effective** remedies and vaccines can be developed.

Finally: The evaluation of all these factors depends inherently on the need for proper monitoring through accurate and wide-spread testing.

And so, for now, the coronavirus has us scratching our collective heads for what long-range effect it will have on individuals and on population life expectancies.

So OK, the race is on to see what kills me, to see what brings that guy with the scythe, the Grim Reaper, to my doorstep first. Who will win, nobody knows … but it should be a close race to the finish. All horses in this race have a chance, and those with the best odds include: Prostate Cancer; Old Age; Coronavirus – all with what I think will go off at about the same 3:1 odds.

There are bunches of other horses, most of them also-rans with poor odds of winning this race – lightning flash, poisonous snake bite, ingesting a toxic mushroom or Yew tree sprig, hit by a car, abducted by aliens, pecked to death by mobbing crows, shot by a jealous husband, and many more. But put all these together into one horse, and maybe that horse would have a slim, very slim, chance.

VII

The Last Nail In the Coffin: And so I am still stuck with the Government Guy's question: "How long has he got left?" What I think is pretty clear, given all the horses that have the best odds – cancer, coronavirus, and old age – I don't have a whole hell of a lot of time left. And at this point, that's all she wrote.

Life Goes On

I

Introduction: I wrote the last chapter (Chapter 34, How Long Has He Got Left?) back in mid-summer 2020. I'm writing this one in mid-summer 2023 – many moons after I'd decided to go off therapy … and let life take care of itself. Well, as they say, lots of water has gone under the bridge since 2020, and as hoped for, life has taken care of itself ... with a few glitches along the way.

II

Cancers A'Plenty: After deciding to go off therapy, my prostate cancer, like a good little bunny, decided to go off into the bushes and not bother me … at least for a while. But there were several other "cancers" lurking in the dark that decided to come out and pester us – while the bunny took his nap.

From out of somewhere far far away, a predator called Covid 19 came a'calling. He crouched in the bushes for a while, measuring his prey, then pounced on us with fangs and claws bared. Killed a million of us in this country alone. But here in the old-folks Co-op, life took care of itself. We all wore masks, stayed out of crowds, got fully vaccinated when it was available, and went on living our lives.

For Sue and me, life actually got better. I wore my masks … because I thought any amount of facial covering helped take away at least some of the uglies. We quit going out for dinner or coffee or entertainment; we stayed home, entertained ourselves, cooked some incredible meals in our own oven … and saved a ton of money.

Finally, I took the jab,[28] not because I thought dying from Covid would be a more terrible way to die than from cancer, but <u>because it would</u> have killed me if there was even a chance that

28 "Jab" is a colloquial term for a vaccine.

I could become the typhoid Mary that infected any one of my family or friends.

And all of us here in the Coop were some of the lucky ones – not one of those million or so in this country who were killed and eaten by the fanged and clawed predator.

III

More Cancers: Meanwhile a more insidious predator lurked within the walls of our co-op building. The company that was supposed to build our complex suddenly went bankrupt, pulled out, and left us in the lurch with a building half-finished.

Shortly after they had pulled the plug on us, I internet-searched the husband-wife team who were principal owners of the bankrupt company … and found them happily at work paving driveways somewhere in Texas. Just another case of an institution (BigBuilders) that was initially set up to serve mankind, ending up with us (mankind) serving it.

And still, life goes on. New workers are found, the building is finished, and we move into our unit in the complex … only to discover a list of improperly installed stuff long enough to fill up all seven of the Dead Sea Scrolls. And boy howdy was it a task to get any of them remedied … but we persisted, and life went on. Until …

Until: About two years after we moved in, a Canada-Cold-Air blast hit us hard, froze and ruptured our (improperly installed) fire sprinkler systems, and flooded eleven individual units plus the community commons area. And then a few years later-on the plumbing in our underground garage began to leak. And so, we've been flooded from above and from below. Noah, where were you when we needed you? God answers: "Next time, fire," says He.

Long story short: The list of institutions that have failed us is long: builders, building inspectors, HUD, roofers, electricians, plumbers, pavers, and installers (of flooring, windows, doors, counter tops, appliances, cupboards, and on and on). Can't tell you how many times we heard: "Sorry but there's nothing we can do about that." And how many times I felt like shouting back: "Maybe if we just followed the money." Ah but…

Ah but: Life goes on. And, as a group of gritty-assed old folks, we've rallied our way through it all – looks like, after fixing and re-installing all the mistakes, we'll have one really decent (and almost totally renovated) living space. With a great new family to enjoy, feast with, laugh along with. And live out our last years with.

IV

Cancer Returns: I've been chemo free for several months now, and the livin' is easy. Shucked all the side effects: chemo brain, joint pain, fatigue, added weight (almost 60 pounds worth), and (some would say unfortunately) my breasts no longer flop and sway when I walk. I can think now, walk in nature almost every day, my writings make sense (to me, anyway), and most of the time I know where I am and where I'm going.

And so, I am a bit jaunty when I go in for my routine MRI … which is where the Wrench-Of-Doom is tossed into my life's pathway. My pelvic lymph nodes are swollen. (So, I'm thinking, *that's* why I've been spending so much time grunting on the crapper. I thought that was just old age, creeping up on me once again.)

Turns out my prostate cancer cells – those devilish, coyote-trickster little bastards – have decided to infiltrate my pelvic lymph nodes … instead of gnawing on the bones of my body, where they were supposed to go. I had steeled myself for the pain and misery of bone fractures, but now I need to think about what to do with a pelvis filled with tumorous lymph nodes.

And so, the decision is made to zap the tumors with radiation and follow up with another round of chemo and ADT (androgen deprivation therapy). Definitely **not** my idea of a fun way to go, but somehow I get talked into it.

Turns out it was worse than not-fun; it was miserable. The pelvic zapping destroyed normal bowel tissues, which led to extreme diarrhea during the 6 weeks of treatment and then for a painfully-long 6 weeks afterwards. Then, the chemo and ADT proved to be times worse than the initial go-around … and so I was an invalid to the treatments once again.

After the treatments were finished, I looked forward to several weeks of recovery (as with the first round) and then to a bit of time with a near-normal body, mind, and soul. But …

But nobody had told me about the possibility of lymphede-ma as a side effect of the radiation, so when my scrotum began to swell, (after a few days of being rather proud of it), I checked back in with the Onc Doc.

She takes a look-see of my scrotum (and to her credit doesn't make a joke about it), says: "Nothing I can do, unless we could try another round of chemo and ADT. There are some new ex-perimental drugs out there. You could go see the urologist, and he might have something."

By this time I have noticed that the lymph swelling has bur-ied my penis … which has made taking a leak a chore of intri-cately excruciating extraction, and, once extraction is completed, holding on for dear life. And so, it's off to the Urologist we go.

Urologist says: "Nothing much I can do. We could do sur-gery, but that doesn't often help. Liposuction would reduce the swelling temporarily, but it just comes back."

I ask: "So where's this going?"

He answers: "Sometimes it can swell to basketball size or even bigger, but usually by then it's too much to handle without painkillers." And I'm thinking: Ah, the miracle of painkillers. Amazing how often they are the first and last line of defense for all sorts of ailments *and* for what the treatments have caused.

And so, wishing someone had warned me of the potential side effects of radiation and wishing even further that since this is a known side effect of radiation, some form of follow-up treat-ment had been developed, Sue and I decide to look into Hospice Care.

V

Looking Back: It's been quite a ride … with all of its ups and downs. We met some wonderful people along the way: doctors, nurses, technicians, receptionists, and more. I loved it when we had time to talk about their lives, their families. I loved it when those talks demonstrated how much they cared about their fam-ilies, their pets, how their kids were doing in school and with their hobbies. All along the way there was the feel of compassion, of deep caring for others, of unbridled love – especially for their patients.

I hate the realization that these profoundly professional and intensely caring caretakers are being herded in one direction by the Barons of BigMed and EvenBiggerOncMed. Herded into protocols prescribed by the trail-boss medical managers who hire the drover doctors to drive the herd along the trail that first-of-all rewards the pharmaceutical companies and their "developments." I hate it that, in order to keep the "cash-cows" moving along, the drovers need to work obscene hours … leaving them with only a few minutes to talk and counsel each individual patient.

I hate it that it is so easy to follow the cattle trail … by simply following the money.

But still … Life Goes On.

Every Life-Journey Different

I

Introduction: It's been said that every life journey is different, and in particular, every cancer patient's experiences while walking the cancer-trail is unique to that individual patient. I am no exception to these axioms, so I present some of my experiences along my cancer-trail as mere observations, certainly not as rules to follow.

II

Truths: I think it is important for an individual to hold certain truths to be self- evident. Among these is the truth that we will all die. As the wag says it: "We're all dying; it's just that some of us are dying faster than others." Since this truth is self-evident, it's time for me to just get on with it.

This getting-on-with-life (while dealing with cancer), has allowed me to be the me I've always wanted (and tried) to be: the happy story-teller able to see the irony, the humor, and the wry-side of life; the family guy who tries to always be there with a nudge of encouragement and a bucket of love; the guy who ain't afraid of nuthin' ... including the real fear of being truly afraid.

It's this last self-truth that has helped me deal with the fear of death and dying. It's also a self-truth that has helped me understand the irony of why – because we are a culture that typically doesn't want to even mention the possibility of death or dying – cancer doctors often feel they need to lie to their patients.

III

More Self-Evident Truths: I hold these truths to be self-evident ... for me: that *movement* is vital for maintaining a vigorously robust mind/body/spirit – that being able to stop, look and learn, listen to, and respect *Nature* is the key to a wholistically healthy existence – that love of and care for *Family* opens the pathway to a lifetime of being pleasurably blessed – that being Creative helps keep our inner juices flowing.

Further, I am convinced that maintaining a *Positive Mental Attitude* and looking on the bright side of life bringeth to the bearer the ascendency of joyful actualization … whereas the strain of lifting and toting all the world's burdens on poor-old-me's-shoulders, and the angst created by the oh-woe-is-me-pity-party mentality – bringeth on even more burden, poverty, and woe.

Finally, after that fateful day of being told I had terminal cancer, I understood from the git-go that I needed to worry through the questions of what do I want, really want? Hopefully, I kept telling myself, I would be able to worry through these questions sometime before my final days.

The *I Want* question, as a matter of principle, includes: what do I want to do; what do I want to *have*; what do I want to *be*?

Interestingly, my *I Wants* were only rarely, if ever, discussed during the visits with my oncology doctors. It seemed as if it was always: here's what *I* (the doctor) *want* to do *for you* (that is: for me). I suppose this is to be expected – from anyone who has signed up to keep patients alive as long as possible and to save as many lives as possible.

I also understand that I was likely a very rare patient who thought that death and dying were natural life events. I was the very rare patient who had lived Life Large – certainly large enough that I didn't need any more time … especially if that time was going to be shrouded in chemo fog and all the other miserable side- effects of the treatments.

I am aware that the Doctor has only been given (by the Medical Management Team that rules the hospital) a few minutes to convince me I need to get on with my treatment … and they don't have time to listen to whatever the hell it is that I want … for Christ's sake.

But dang it, this whole setup seems to me to be very un-holistic. And so, I go on my own little way of finding and trying to achieve *My* wants list.

IV

What Do I Want To Do: After the cancer diagnosis, I spent considerable time and effort muddling around with this question, and finally decided on this: What I want to do is spend whatever amount of time I have left (at the onset, this could have been less than 5 months or maybe up to about 5 years) doing the four things (my Self-Evident Truths) that I think are important: Moving; In Nature; with Family; and finally, taking a stab at being Creative.

What I've found, after five years of trying to do just this, is that this four-legged approach, on a daily basis, has been overwhelmingly satisfying ... for me. Those days when I'd given all of my four legs at least a smidgen of attention, I'd feel like I'd actually accomplished something. And, having accomplished something, I had hope that tomorrow might be an even better day.

I've also found that I might be able to wobble along on three of the legs for maybe a day or two. For example: I might not have enough juice to get out and walk, or chemo fog might have me so befuddled I couldn't come up with even one coherent sentence to put down on paper. And still, by limping along on three legs, I could persist.

But, after that third or fourth day on three legs, I'd feel like I'd be better off calling in the guy with the scythe.

So, being an old creature with cancer, hobbling along on four legs has worked for me. But, inherent in the, "working for me," is that I have been fortunate enough to have done almost everything I ever wanted to do. So, when asked: "Wouldn't you want to do this or that, go hither or thither, wander yonder and beyond ?" I can honestly answer, "Been there; done that."

Point being that while, "Living Life Large and doing whatever felt like fun and whatever would bring me joy at the time," has a hell of a lot of downsides, it surely shortens your end-of-life "bucket list." At least it did for me.

V

What Do I Want To Have: I hold this truth to be self-evident – that I have, and have always had, everything I've ever needed … certainly everything I've needed to stay alive. Elsewise, I wouldn't be here now, would I?

I've been around a lot of rich people, and most of them are as miserable as sin. Evidently, wanting to have it all digests into "I know having all this (money or power or whatever) will only make me sicker, but I'm going to devour as much of it as I possibly can anyway."

Telling comment from our Hospice Nurse when I asked which patients she found the most difficult to deal with; her answer: "those rich folks who have no one. All alone in their huge mansions, they're so terribly lonesome."

I, on the other hand, finally got the one remaining wish I'd always jokingly asked Santa for: a Ferrari. Kris, our oldest, presented me with one shortly after I got cancer – such a nice gift. It's a red and white and black racing model, about 7 1/2 inches long, remote controlled and battery driven. It's a hoot to whip it around in circles on our floor. Initially we had it parked in the display case our grandson (and Kris' son), Bret, had built for us, but the great-grandkids' photos accumulated and pushed it out to its current parking spot.

Ah well – possessions are just that: now you have them; now you don't.

VI

What Do I Want To Be: This is perhaps the toughest question of all – because it will force me to think about how I want to live my life … from now on. It makes no sense for me to try to rely on the any of the titles I've achieved to offer any form of solace now; no sense to rest on any of the (very few) laurels I've accumulated to make me happy today; no sense to polish any of the (even fewer) trophies I've won, expecting them to add brightness to my day.

The real rewards in life come from working toward creating positive inner outcomes (haves) such as: happiness, joy, hope, love, trust, passion, compassion, enthusiasm, astonishment, serenity, gratitude, interest, amusement, awe, inspiration, and more.

In other words, what I want to *be* is someone who is actively working toward *having* those attributes that create positive inner outcomes. It's all in the *doing*. What I want to *do* is whatever it takes to bring about happiness (or any of the other positive mental/emotional outcomes), whatever it takes to *have* a happy life … so that I can *be* truly happy.

VII

How Do I Do My Daily Do-Its: Sue and I rise with the sun – or when our bladders tell us to. (We chucked the alarm clocks long ago… because we are old now.) We plan our walks around several variables: the weather; Sue's busy schedule; and my current state of "body-juice," which is usually OK *if* I'm not on chemo drugs at the time.

We have a dozen or so sidewalk trails we can saunter along, treks that range from about a mile to just over two miles long. Most of our trails, even though they are in the middle of suburbia, take us by some favorite bird-watching or small critter-spotting areas.

We plan breakfast and lunch around the time when we walk – during summer heat, that means a very early morning walk; perhaps mid to late afternoon in winter; maybe sometime closer to noon during milder weather.

We eat damned well – as they say: living high on the hog – mostly organic or local-grown foods. Big no-nos are anything highly processed or overly sugared or that contains preservatives or artificial flavors or colors. (One exception is the lushly salty-tasty ridgie-style potato chips – because everyone needs to struggle with at least one food-vice.)

BC (Before Cancer) we were mostly vegetarians, but ACD (After Cancer Diagnosis) we added some occasional red meat – because I wanted to give my bones and red blood cells the best chance possible to keep on growing.

All this, of course, relies on an in-house chief chef (Sue) who can do the dinner fixings from scratch ... and she is a champ of a cook. The only art-form I am competent in is food prep – I am Chef Sue's Sous Chef: for breakfast, I slice the tomatoes and avocados, cut the bread, and grind the coffee beans. For a very short time I tried being chief chef for just one dinner a week, but I was soon fired – total incompetence was only one of the major complaints.

After breakfast, I retire to my office for my attempt at creativity; Sue is busy as gardener, Secretary of the Branchwood Village Board (now retired), chief chef and housekeeper, family matron, and my caretaker. ("She can cook and sew and make flowers grow, and she understands my pain." Bob Dylan)

In my office I am literally surrounded by artifacts of and from Nature: pictures of animals and animal fetishes, rocks and gemstones collected from here and there, plants that Sue is mothering, dream catchers, sachets and tied bundles of sage, lavender, and other herbs, found-feathers, deer antlers, bison horns, and more.

My routine is to dab some essential oil of sage on forehead (third eye), sternum (also known as the "Breastplate of Righteousness), and inner wrists (acupuncture site of Pericardium-6, a site that is supposed to exert an effect on the body's chi). Since we are a non-smoking building, I use the oil instead of a smudge.

Properly anointed, I do a few minutes of shamanic drumming to the four directions. I drum because it's a routine that gets me off my duff and into my Chair-of-Creativity ... and because it gives me a chance to give thanks, and it seems to elevate my overall sense of well-being. Recently, scientists have discovered that repetitive drumming alters certain brain-wave frequencies – which might explain why my writings often seem so creatively crazy-assed. (The moving finger writes; and, having writ, moves on ...)

Once seated, I try to write for at least a few hours, and during the day, I try to fulfill the six necessities of being a writer: I read, read, read, and I write, write, write.

Breaks for coffee (and to get rid of the coffee) require walking among our household ecosystem of ambience that Sue has created: artworks of animals and nature; photo walls of Sue and my parents and grandparents, of Sue and I with our kids as they are growing up, of our kids and their kids as they are living their lives, and of our grandkids' kids as they are growing up, getting married and creating our great grandkids ... the kids who occupy the final wall.

A few years back our kids gave us one of those photo and video thingies (a Photo Spring), and it sits smack dab in the middle of our home, right where you can't get anywhere without walking by it. Family members from near and far have sent photos and videos of what's happening in their lives.

And so, Sue and I have, over the years, spent long hours standing there watching the family's antics, celebrations, and pratfalls. Our kids and grandkids have also been great about calling, sending emails, and occasionally stopping by for a brief visit.

All this adds up to what feels as if a galaxy-sized mist of stardust has been tossed our way to brighten our lives. It's this brightness that Sue and I talk about a lot – often several times a day (between my naps) we sit and talk, remembering the good times, trying to recollect what that person's name was or exactly where it was that this or that funny thing happened.

And we talk about how this has been the biggest blessing ever – how we've been able to have the time to sit and talk about our lives gone past; about how our families are living their lives now; about how we plan to live whatever time we have left together … all this brought to us along with the blessing of a cancer diagnosis.

The Great Mystery

I

The Great Mystery: Many Native Americans believe that death places you in the hands of the Great Mystery. The Great Mystery (also known as Wakan Tanka, or the Great Spirit, or The One Above, and a variety of other names) is a term used to describe the sacred or the divine, and it can be interpreted as the power or sacredness that resides in everything – every plant and tree and waterway and mountain and rock … and every creature (even including those upright, two-legged human creatures).

Death, then, puts you in direct touch with all the spirits of the world – you become an integrated part of all that is sacred or divine. In other words, you become a spiritual partner with everything and everyone in the world. For me, thinking of it this way means that, as death reveals the Great Mystery, that revelation brings with it a new learning, as well as a new reckoning.

I remember Sue and I were honored by being invited to attend a Pow Wow at Haskell University, a celebration of the next path a particular seeker of the Great Mystery would be taking. All the celebrants were invited to dance and sing to the beat of the drum, rhythmically in tune with the heart's pulse. The seeker, a patient with terminal cancer, sat proudly at the seat of honor during the entire Pow Wow.

For me it was an eye-opener for how we could think about and for how we could approach death.

II

The Afterlife: You can argue for an afterlife if you want to. (I'd want to come back as a quartzite rock that is sturdy-hard immune to all the cancers our species, in its infinite wisdom, has brought to this world.)

Or you could believe that you'd end up amongst a cuddle-huddle of 72 vestal virgins. (Would be just my luck that all of them would have chosen to honor their vow of chastity.)

Or you might be trying for a heavenly reward instead of the fire below … or even worse, the purgatory of not knowing exactly where the hell you were … or where the hell you were going.

Or you might believe, as I do, that when it's over, it's over. No big fanfare, no meet-up with St. Peter, no enclave of virgins more interested in tending the fire on Vesta's altar … than in taking care of moi, the newly departed. Dust return-eth to dust.

We tend to want to put our own spin on what will happen to us after death. But the truth is that no one really knows. You can stir the embers of your inner shadow all you want … and you still won't be certain where the after-death fates will take you.

After death is not my biggest concern; how to approach death, and how to think about death have become my bigger concerns. Big enough concerns to dominate my everyday worries. And I agree that looking forward to having the Great Mystery finally revealed is one good way to approach death.

III

Dying With Grace: I read an article a while back, written by a daughter whose father, a medical doctor, was dying from cancer. He confided to her that all he really wanted to do was to die with grace. That one really got me to thinking. What exactly is grace? How do you make yourself "full of grace?" How do you die, embracing grace?

I get the idea that dying from cancer is never the most graceful of ways to depart this world – lots of pain and suffering and humiliatingly awful stuff like incontinence, loss of bowel control, cognitive decline, falling down and unable to get back up.

In Christian terms grace can be defined as "God's favor toward the unworthy," or "God's benevolence on the undeserving." In other words, in His grace, God is willing to forgive and bless us despite the fact that we fall short of living righteously. Well, I'll be damned – cancer sure looks to me like it's a hell of a way to show forgiveness … even though I will admit that I have my share of stuff that needs forgiving.

But I don't think the good doctor in the article meant it that way. I think he meant that he wanted to die without stumbling and fumbling and bumbling all over himself. I think that he was worried, as a doctor, that becoming less graceful as a person would make him seem less professional, perhaps less a man, especially to his family. At least that's how I feel, how I worry about my final days and how they will leave an impression on those I love.

It's that prolonging of the messiness of dying that makes contemplating death such a difficult task for many of us to bear. How will the way I handle my own death appear to those around me? How ungraceful will my actions be, and thus how ungraceful will the memories of me be?

IV

How Fast, Death? For me there is the distinct contrast between the two extremes: 1) the profound blessing of being given the time to discuss the life I have lived with my family and loved ones – a life full of great joy and satisfaction, some hilarious moments worth laughing about even now, and, yes, some times of grief and sorrow, played against the contrast of: 2) the fear that, if it takes too long to die, my body will finally rebel and turn me into a physically graceless buffoon.

I think of those we knew who died suddenly. Sue's dad came home from a round of golf – his lifetime favorite hobby – told Dorothy (his wife and Sue's mom) that he was tired, went into the living room, sat down to rest in his favorite easy chair … and never got up.

Similar thing happened to two of our neighbors – each of them discovered her husband on the floor, dead. And there's another neighbor, a fellow prostate cancer sufferer who went to hospice only a few months after diagnosis. He deteriorated quickly and was being attended to as a dying man when … he suddenly sat up in bed and asked, "What's going on here?" One of the attending nurses answered, "Well, you're dying." And he laid back down and died.

My dad died suddenly: While flying a National Guard plane, a wingtip gas tank broke loose, tore off the plane's tail assembly (making it impossible to control up or down), and he went almost straight down … to his grave, as they say. Gravity working on a heavy metal tomb … with a still-alive human-being strapped inside.

I worry about those last few moments he lived through. If the tail was torn off at 10,000 feet, his trajectory to the ground would take approximately 30 seconds; about a minute or so from somewhere around 15,000 feet; maybe a minute and a half if he'd been able to climb to 20,000 feet.

Later, when I was talking with Gen. Clark, his flying partner that day and his commanding officer, the general said it simply: "We were flying a tandem, climbing up out of Lockbourne Air Force Base. We went into a cloud bank together … and when we came out, his plane was nowhere to be seen. Going into that cloud bank was the last I saw of your dad."

Free falling objects reach terminal velocity, about 120 mph, in roughly 12 seconds. According to newspaper reports, my dad's crash site was not scattered, not much bigger than the plane itself. His plane likely went into a spin, possibly an upside-down spin, and corkscrewed straight down into the ground ... at somewhere around 200 mph.

To this day I wonder what he thought about during those last few seconds. How did he physically react to the frantic despair of the moment? What did he exclaim, what words did he shout out … if any? So young, he may have never given death a second thought. Or WWII might have permanently etched the possibility of dying into the depths of his brain's amygdala … and he had chosen to, at least for the most part, ignore the etchings.

I am very certain that, as an instructor pilot, he did everything he could to right the plane – an impossible task without the tail gear. And that might have been all he had time for – a monumental physical struggle.

Recent research indicates that our brains may actually flash our lives before us right before we die. If there was time for that flash in my dad's brain, I only hope he was shown the good stuff I'd done; not the dumb and dumber stuff … because to this day, I realize he tried very hard to be a good father to me and to my sisters. (In my case, as the saying goes: You can only work with the soil you are given.)

V

Animal Grace: The doctor's story in the magazine included his two hunting dogs and how he treasured his time working with them. There is nothing more graceful than a working animal, doing the job it was meant to do. Nothing in this world is graceful enough that it can give a more profound sense of awe. At the same time, dogs are notorious for, well, for being dogs. Their screw-ups can be colossal, as in: "Oops, boss, I probably shouldn't have chased that skunk. But it sure looked like fun at the time."

And thus, it takes a person full of grace (in the sense of having mercy on those that may not always perform in ways worthy of merit) to be a decent trainer of dogs (or, for that matter, to work "decently or gracefully" with any of our domesticated animals).

In this story of the dying doctor, it is impressive that a more profound sense of grace is relayed through the doctor's work with his dogs ... rather than through the clients he had treated daily in his profession. But this is often the case with people who are intimately connected with nature – with the tame and the wild animals, and with the plants on the land, and with the mountains on the horizon.

And finally, the magazine story does not tell us whether or not the doctor died grace-fully. We are left to guess at his physical suffering ... or lack of it. What we see, instead, is that, after he dies, his daughter (and writer of the piece) takes the dogs for a run – savoring those moments with the dogs, reflections of the training her father left behind as a part of his legacy.

VI

Nature's Grace: Aldo Leopold in his book, Sand County Almanac, talks about watching a creature die. He looks into the wolf's eyes he has just shot, watching the fierce green fire in her eyes ... as the fire goes out. Still in his youth, Leopold had his reasons for hunting, but while he watches the dying fire in the wolf's eyes, he realizes that the wolf has a different reasoning about being made into a preyed-upon animal.

In Leopold's story, not only the wolf, but also the mountain the wolf came from, had differing reasons for wanting and for needing to remain alive. And those reasons were interlaced with each other – wolf and mountain interactions helped keep each other more alive … which then made it more possible for mankind to be more alive.

Fire, to glowing ember, to ash; the heated aura of fierce green fire, to a now-flaccid orb, shrinking into the orbit of an overcast cloudiness. All this in turn leading to Leopold's epiphany that we are all connected – wolves and mountains, us and the wolves, and us and the mountains.

Shakespeare said that the eyes are the window into the soul. As a veterinarian, there were many times when I watched death as its story of the-window-into-the-soul was played out before me.

There were times when I would watch as an animal's spirit and soul-life were slowly ebbing away, gradually leaving behind a window scarred by the sands of time. One or more of the chronic diseases – or just plain old age – were creeping into his everyday experience.

Typically, the animal's "window into his soul" would reflect his inability to reconcile physical problems such as: incontinence, organ systems gone bad, legs that could carry the load no more – any one of these concerns a major impact on what that animal viewed as his necessary contribution to his human family.

Oftentimes clients would also notice the eye's clouding over and would tell me: "Doc, I don't think he's there anymore. I don't feel like he sees me or anything else now. It's so sad." And I would know it was time to gently suggest: "Perhaps it's time to relieve him of his suffering. Maybe we should consider euthanasia."

On the one hand, I hated "putting animals to sleep" – and what a nice, gentle euphemism that is. On the other hand, I understood, from somewhere deep within, that the pains of living had overwhelmed the creature's will or the ability to live any longer.

And so, for me it was a duty to be endured, a task that required a steely distancing so the job would be done efficiently. Sometimes the pet's parents wanted to watch; sometimes not. The watchers were inevitably surprised at the suddenness and completeness of death – as the plunger of the syringe is pushed, and the injection is still moving into the vein, one huge inhale and then collapse. Many broke into tears. And I would struggle to remain professionally detached.

The observation that gives me solace – and other veterinarians have said the same thing was true for them – is that many of the euthanized would take that one last huge breath, look up into my eyes, and their eyes would tell me what a relief they felt.

VII

Last Words: Perhaps this is Nature's way of accepting the finality of death, Nature's way of accepting the final journey that carries us into the realm of the Great Mystery. Nature's way of reuniting our spirit with the soul of Nature.

Acknowledgments

Writers draw strength and inspirations from many sources, and I'd like to acknowledge three statements of belief that have formed the foundation of my approach to Nature Walking With Cancer.

"In the beginning of all things, wisdom and knowledge were the animals; for Tirawa, the One Above, did not speak directly to man. He sent the animals to tell man that he showed himself through the beasts, and that from them, and from the stars and the sun and the moon, man should learn." —*Chief Latakots-Lesa, Pawnee Tribe*

"We believe that the domestic animals were sent here to accept the diseases of humans...and to show them how to heal these diseases." —*Tis Mal Crow, Native American "Root Doctor"*

"If there were no plants we would not be here. We breathe in what they breathe out. That is how we learn from them."
—*Keetoowah, Cherokee Teacher*

I would also like to thank my hundreds of four-legged patients for their role as my teachers. My wife Sue is my strength, my way of staying rooted to the wellness that comes from our Earth Mother. To my family and friends who read and listened to my stories and laughed, or cried. Finally, I'd like to thank the folks at Anamcara Press for their editorial input and for giving my story a voice.

About The Author

R andy Kidd, D.V.M., Ph.D. holds doctorates in Veterinary Medicine from The Ohio State University and Veterinary and Clinical Pathology from Kansas State University. After practicing traditional veterinary medicine for many years, he opened Honoring the Animals, a holistic practice in Kansas City, Missouri. Dr. Kidd was the author of two books including "Dr Kidd's Guide to Herbal Care For Dogs," a columnist for multiple pet care magazines including Dogs Naturally and Herbs for Health. He was Past President of the American Holistic Veterinary Medical Association and a leader in many other civic and nature-oriented organizations. Retired from active practice, he continued writing, speaking and teaching on the big topic of "Reuniting The Human Spirit With The Soul Of Nature." And just like a rabbit playing tricks, he died on January 15, 2024, toward the end of the Year of the Rabbit!

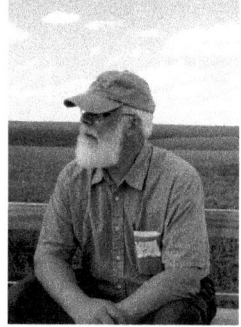

www.ingramcontent.com/pod-product-compliance
Lightning Source LLC
Chambersburg PA
CBHW062122020426
42335CB00013B/1060